Analgesia and Pain Management

Guest Editor

JOANNE PAUL-MURPHY, DVM, Dipl. ACZM

VETERINARY CLINICS OF NORTH AMERICA: EXOTIC ANIMAL PRACTICE

www.vetexotic.theclinics.com

Consulting Editor
AGNES E. RUPLEY, DVM, Dipl. ABVP–Avian

January 2011 • Volume 14 • Number 1

SAUNDERS an imprint of ELSEVIER, Inc.

W.B. SAUNDERS COMPANY

A Division of Elsevier Inc.

1600 John F. Kennedy Boulevard • Suite 1800 • Philadelphia, Pennsylvania 19103-2899

http://www.vetexotic.theclinics.com

VETERINARY CLINICS OF NORTH AMERICA: EXOTIC ANIMAL PRACTICE Volume 14, Number 1
January 2011 ISSN 1094-9194, ISBN-13: 978-1-4557-0520-7

Editor: John Vassallo; j.vassallo@elsevier.com
Developmental Editor: Jessica Demetriou

Veterinary Clinics of North America: Exotic Animal Practice (ISSN 1094-9194) is published in January, May, and September by Elsevier, Inc., 360 Park Avenue South, New York, NY 10010-1710. Subscription prices are $212.00 per year for US individuals, $345.00 per year for US institutions, $108.00 per year for US students and residents, $253.00 per year for Canadian individuals, $407.00 per year for Canadian institutions, $285.00 per year for international individuals, $407.00 per year for international institutions and $139.00 per year for Canadian and foreign students/residents. To receive student/resident rate, orders must be accompanied by name of affiliated institution, date of term, and the *signature* of program/residency coordinator on institution letterhead. Orders will be billed at individual rate until proof of status is received. Foreign air speed delivery is included in all *Clinics* subscription prices. All prices are subject to change without notice. **POSTMASTER:** Send address changes to *Veterinary Clinics of North America: Exotic Animal Practice*, Elsevier Health Sciences Division, Subscription Customer Service, 3251 Riverport Lane, Maryland Heights, MO 63043. **Customer Service: Telephone: 1-800-654-2452** (U.S. and Canada); **1-314-447-8871** (outside U.S. and Canada). **Fax: 1-314-447-8029.** E-mail: journalscustomerservice-usa@elsevier.com (for print support); journalsonlinesupport-usa@elsevier.com (for online support).

Reprints. For copies of 100 or more of articles in this publication, please contact the Commercial Reprints Department, Elsevier Inc., 360 Park Avenue South, New York, New York 10010-1710. Tel.: (212)-633-3813; Fax: (212)-633-1935; E-mail: reprints@elsevier.com.

Veterinary Clinics of North America: Exotic Animal Practice is covered in *MEDLINE/PubMed (Index Medicus)*.

Printed and bound by CPI Group (UK) Ltd, Croydon, CR0 4YY

Transferred to Digital Print 2011

Contributors

CONSULTING EDITOR

AGNES E. RUPLEY, DVM
Diplomate, American Board of Veterinary Practitioners-Avian Practice; Director
and Chief Veterinarian, All Pets Medical and Laser Surgical Center, College Station, Texas

GUEST EDITOR

JOANNE PAUL-MURPHY, DVM
Diplomate, American College of Zoological Medicine; Professor, Companion Zoological
Animals, Department of Medicine and Epidemiology, School of Veterinary Medicine,
University of California Davis, Davis, California

AUTHORS

LINDA S. BARTER, MVSc, PhD
Diplomate, American College of Veterinary Anesthesiologists; Assistant Professor,
Anesthesiology, Department of Surgical and Radiological Sciences, School
of Veterinary Medicine, University of California Davis, Davis, California

SHERRY K. COX, MS, PhD
Clinical Associate Professor, Department of Comparative Medicine, College
of Veterinary Medicine, University of Tennessee, Knoxville, Tennessee

MICHELLE G. HAWKINS, VMD
Diplomate, American Board of Veterinary Practitioners-Avian Practice; Associate
Professor, Companion Zoological Animals, Department of Medicine and Epidemiology,
School of Veterinary Medicine, University of California Davis, Davis, California

MATTHEW S. JOHNSTON, VMD
Diplomate, American Board of Veterinary Practitioners-Avian Practice; Department of
Clinical Sciences, College of Veterinary Medicine and Biomedical Sciences, Colorado
State University, Fort Collins, Colorado

MARILYN A. KOSKI, DVM
Staff Veterinarian, Companion Avian and Exotic Pet Medicine Wellness Service;
Staff Veterinarian, Small and Exotic Animal Acupuncture Service, University of California,
Veterinary Medical Teaching Hospital, Davis, California

BUTCH KUKANICH, DVM, PhD
Diplomate, American College of Veterinary Clinical Pharmacology; Associate Professor,
College of Veterinary Medicine, Kansas State University, Manhattan, Kansas

AMY L. MILLER, PhD
Research Associate, Institute of Neuroscience; Comparative Biology Centre, Medical
School, Newcastle University, Newcastle upon Tyne, United Kingdom

CRAIG MOSLEY, DVM, MSc
Diplomate, American College of Veterinary Anesthesiologists; Director of Anesthesia Services, Department of Anesthesia, Canada West Veterinary Specialists, Vancouver, British Columbia, Canada

JOANNE PAUL-MURPHY, DVM
Diplomate, American College of Zoological Medicine; Professor, Companion Zoological Animals, Department of Medicine and Epidemiology, School of Veterinary Medicine, University of California Davis, Davis, California

CLAIRE A. RICHARDSON, BVM&S, MRCVS
Veterinary Surgeon, Institute of Neuroscience; Comparative Biology Centre, Medical School, Newcastle University, Newcastle upon Tyne, United Kingdom

NARDA G. ROBINSON, DO, DVM, MS
Department of Clinical Sciences, Center for Comparative and Integrative Pain Medicine, Colorado State University, Fort Collins, Colorado

JESSICA K. RYCHEL, DVM
Department of Clinical Sciences, Center for Comparative and Integrative Pain Medicine, Colorado State University, Fort Collins, Colorado

NICO J. SCHOEMAKER, DVM, PhD
Diplomate, European College of Zoological Medicine (Small Mammal & Avian), Diplomate, American Board of Veterinary Practitioners-Avian Practice; Department of Clinical Sciences of Companion Animals, Faculty of Veterinary Medicine, Utrecht University, Utrecht, The Netherlands

MARCY J. SOUZA, DVM, MPH
Diplomate, American Board of Veterinary Practitioners-Avian Practice; Diplomate, American College of Veterinary Preventive Medicine; Assistant Professor, Department of Comparative Medicine, College of Veterinary Medicine, University of Tennessee, Knoxville, Tennessee

CRAIG W. STEVENS, PhD
Professor of Pharmacology, Department of Pharmacology & Physiology, Oklahoma State University-Center for Health Sciences, Tulsa, Oklahoma

JOOST J. UILENREEF, DVM, MVR
Diplomate, European College of Veterinary Anaesthesia and Analgesia, Department of Clinical Sciences of Companion Animals, Faculty of Veterinary Medicine, Utrecht University, Utrecht, The Netherlands

HUGO van OOSTROM, DVM, PhD
Department of Clinical Sciences of Companion Animals, Faculty of Veterinary Medicine, Utrecht University, Utrecht, The Netherlands

E. SCOTT WEBER III, VMD, MSc (Distinction) Aquatic Pathobiology/Veterinary Science
Associate Professor of Clinical Aquatic Animal Medicine, Department of Medicine and Epidemiology, School of Veterinary Medicine, University of California Davis, Davis, California

Contents

The treatment and prevention of pain in zoologic companion animals is difficult because of the lack of data available on the safety and efficacy of analgesics. Pharmacokinetic (PK)-pharmacodynamic (PD) studies integrate changes in drug concentrations and changes in the drug's effect. All experimental studies assessing the PDs of analgesics have limitations in animals, but the data provided by experimental studies are valuable in designing dosages. Placebo-controlled, randomized, and blinded clinical trials provide the best PK and PD data, but are rarely performed in major veterinary species because of the number of animals required for the study, lack of preliminary PK and PD data in a given species, species-specific differences in PK and PD, and ethical and toxicologic concerns. The usefulness and limitations as well as considerations for interpreting PK, PD, and controlled clinical studies are discussed. An example of allometric analysis of buprenorphine in mammals is also included.

The increasing use of fish resources and a greater understanding of aquatic animal medicine demands providing evidence-based veterinary care for these animals. Because fish are aquatic as well as being pokilothermic, there are several unique anatomic and physiologic considerations that must be understood when working with these animals. Veterinarians need to adapt methodologies for examining, performing diagnostics, and treating fish patients to decrease stress, decrease fear, and avoid and/or decrease nociception. This article briefly defines stress, reviews and compares fish neuroanatomic pathways associated with nociception, discusses behavioral observations, summarizes current use of analgesics for fish patients, and concludes with the ongoing controversy regarding pain on this topic.

Preclinical studies of analgesia in amphibians or recommendations for clinical use of analgesics in amphibian species are extremely limited. This article briefly reviews the issues surrounding the use of analgesics in amphibians, starting with common definitions of pain and analgesia when applied to nonhuman animals. Nociceptive and endogenous opioid systems in amphibians are reviewed, and results of preclinical research on opioid and nonopioid analgesics summarized. Recommended opioid and nonopioid analgesics are summarized, and practical recommendations made for their clinical use.

The ability of reptiles to "feel" pain and the significance of pain or nociception on physiologic homeostasis is an exceedingly complex question requiring integration of both physiologic and behavioral evidence. Until further information is available, it would seem most ethical for veterinarians to assume that reptiles are capable of feeling pain, and to treat or manage pain when there is reasonable evidence that pain is present. With increased information available regarding analgesic use in reptiles and with the heightened awareness of the importance of analgesia for zoologic companion animals, it is likely that more veterinarians will provide pain relief to their reptile patients.

Avian analgesia is now recognized as a critical component of avian medicine and surgery. The need to recognize pain and to provide pain relief is the first step, and many anecdotal therapeutic doses have been extrapolated from other companion animals. Several published research investigations, using several species of birds, have begun to provide avian analgesia therapeutic information for clinical application. The challenge is to continue pushing this research forward with appreciation that there are approximately 10,000 known species of birds, perhaps 200 species commonly kept as pets, and that each species has a range of behaviors as varied as their species-specific PKs and PDs to each analgesic drug.

Rodents of all species are frequently kept as companion animals, with increasing client expectations for the care of their animals. Fortunately, specialist veterinary interest and information is now available for treatment of rodents. In the field of rodent analgesia particularly, much can be learned from the methods developed for preventing and alleviating pain in animals undergoing research studies in laboratories throughout the world. This article reviews advances in pain detection techniques in rodents and makes recommendations on analgesic agents that are available for the alleviation of pain.

With the increasing popularity of rabbits as household pets, the complexity of diagnostic and surgical procedures performed on rabbits is increasing, along with the frequency of routine surgical procedures. More practitioners are faced with the need to provide adequate analgesia for this species. Preemptive analgesia prior to planned surgical interventions may reduce nervous system changes in response to noxious input, as well as reduce postoperative pain levels and analgesic drug requirements. Concurrent administration of analgesic drugs to anesthetized rabbits undergoing painful procedures is warranted both pre- and intraoperatively as well as postoperatively. This article discusses the neuropharmacologic and pharmacologic aspects of pain in rabbits, and reviews current protocols for the use of analgesic drugs.

The growing popularity of ferrets as pets has created the demand for advanced veterinary care for these patients. Pain is associated with a broad range of conditions, including acute or chronic inflammatory disease, neoplasia, and trauma, as well as iatrogenic causes, such as surgery and diagnostic procedures. Effective pain management requires knowledge and skills to assess pain, good understanding of the pathophysiology of pain, and general knowledge of pharmacologic and pharmacodynamic principles. Unfortunately, scientific studies on efficacy, pharmacokinetics, pharmacodynamics, and safety of analgesic drugs in the ferret are limited. However, basic rules on the treatment of pain and mechanisms of action, safety, and efficacy of analgesic drugs in other species can be adapted and applied to pain management in ferrets. This article aims to make an inventory of what is known on the recognition of pain in ferrets, what analgesic drugs are currently used in ferrets, and how they can be adopted in a patient-orientated pain management plan to provide effective pain relief while reducing and monitoring for unwanted side effects.

Numerous analgesics are available for use in animals, but only a few have been used or studied in zoologic species. Tramadol is a relatively new analgesic that is available in an inexpensive, oral form, and is not controlled. Studies examining the effect of tramadol in zoologic species suggest that significant differences exist in pharmacokinetics parameters as well as analgesic dynamics. This article reviews the current literature on the use of tramadol in humans, domestic animals, and zoologic species.

Injury and illness in zoologic companion animals can lead to significant pain and debilitation. Recovery can be slow and sometimes frustrating. By augmenting recovery from trauma or disease with physical medicine and rehabilitation techniques, recovery can be more rapid and complete. Physical medicine techniques, such as massage, can augment recovery from a painful injury or surgery by reducing edema, improving postoperative ileus, and decreasing anxiety. Familiarity with the tools of rehabilitation along with focus on pain management, strengthening, and proprioception improve patient care.

Research in complementary and alternative veterinary medicine (CAVM) has increased dramatically in recent years. Acupuncture represents the most commonly practiced and extensively researched of all the CAVM modalities. Acupuncture is considered a valid therapeutic mode of treatment that can be integrated into Western veterinary medicine for the treatment of large, small, and zoological companion animal patients, especially in the area of analgesia. This article is intended to provide a guide for the zoological companion animal practitioner to gain a basic understanding of acupuncture and its potential for use in the zoological companion animal patient.

THE CLINICS ARE NOW AVAILABLE ONLINE!

Access your subscription at:
www.theclinics.com

FORTHCOMING ISSUES

May 2011
The Exotic Animal Respiratory System
Cathy Johnson-Delaney, DVM,
DABVP-Avian, DABVP-Exotic Companion
Mammal, and Susan E. Orosz, PhD, DVM,
DABVP-Avian, DECAMS, Guest Editors

September 2011
Zoonoses, Public Health and the Exotic
Animal Practitioner
Marcy J. Souza, DVM, MPH, DABVP-Avian,
Guest Editor

RECENT ISSUES

September 2010
Advances and Updates in Internal Medicine
Kemba Marshall, DVM, DABVP-Avian,
Guest Editor

May 2010
Endoscopy and Endosurgery
Stephen J. Divers, BVetMed, DZooMed,
DACZM, DipECAMS(herp), FRCVS,
Guest Editor

January 2010
Bariatrics
Sherman M. Hooper, DVM,
Diol ABVP—Avian, and
Patricia Gray, DVM, MS, Guest Editors

RELATED INTEREST

Veterinary Clinics of North America: Small Animal Practice (Volume 38, Issue 6,
November 2008)
Updates in Pain Management
Karol A. Mathews, DVM, DVSc, Guest Editor

THE CLINICS ARE NOW AVAILABLE ONLINE!

Access your subscription at:
www.theclinics.com

Erratum

In the September 2010 issue, on the Contributors page, the diplomate statuses of two authors were interchanged. The correct author information is as follows:

Olivier Taeymans, DVM, PhD
Diplomate, European College of Veterinary Diagnostic Imaging; Assistant Professor of Diagnostic Imaging, Department of Clinical Sciences, Tufts University Cummings School of Veterinary Medicine, North Grafton, Massachusetts

Robert Wagner, VMD
Diplomate, American Board of Veterinary Practitioners-Exotic Companion Mammal Practice; Associate Professor of Medicine, University of Pittsburgh, Division of Laboratory Animal Services, University of Pittsburgh, Pittsburgh, Pennsylvania

Vet Clin Exot Anim 14 (2011) xi
doi:10.1016/j.cvex.2010.10.001
1094-9194/11/$ — see front matter © 2011 Elsevier Inc. All rights reserved.
vetexotic.theclinics.com

Preface

Analgesia and Pain Management

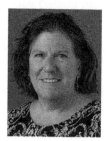

Joanne Paul-Murphy, DVM, DACZM
Guest Editor

I was honored to be asked to be the guest editor for the second analgesia edition of the *Veterinary Clinics of North America: Exotic Animal Practice*. In 2001, the first publication combined analgesia with anesthesia, both very important topics in zoological companion animal medicine at that time. Analgesia has emerged and separated from anesthesia as a critical issue in veterinary care and has unique challenges for zoological companion animal medicine and surgery. The concern for animal welfare has heightened our awareness that pain can be harmful to animals and thus the mitigation and prevention of pain are crucial. Chronic pain can adversely affect an animal's well-being, affecting the health-related quality of life. In zoological medicine the term "chronic" and "quality of life" are relative to the life span of the species, which can range from a few years to several decades. All animals, from octopi to birds, reptiles to mammals, possess the neuroanatomic and neuropharmacologic components necessary for the transduction, transmission, and perception of noxious stimuli. The issue of when does nociception become pain still plagues the evaluation of fish, amphibian, and reptile analgesia studies. The future direction of analgesia investigations must consider the comparative aspects among various species, beginning with the basic assumption that animals feel pain.

Each article in this issue examines the current metrics and research techniques applied to domestic animal pain and treatment, and which techniques can be cross-applied to investigate similar concerns in companion zoological animals.

This new edition provides the most current information on therapies and techniques to reduce pain in zoological species. In each of the reviews, the authors discuss the challenges of recognizing painful behaviors in the particular species they are writing about. Even if we as caregivers could recognize when zoological companion animals are in pain, we are further challenged by the knowledge that species variation is tremendous and the extrapolation of what limited information is available is sometimes insufficient to address the individual animal's need for pain relief.

Vet Clin Exot Anim 14 (2011) xiii–xvi
doi:10.1016/j.cvex.2010.10.002
1094-9194/11/$ – see front matter © 2011 Elsevier Inc. All rights reserved.

The first article provides a primer on pharmacokinetic and pharmacodynamic approaches to understanding analgesic therapy, independent of species. Dr Butch KuKanich provides insight into the different types of research studies and clinical recommendations for analgesia therapy in zoological companion animals. His expertise in clinical pharmacology and interest in zoological medicine is presented in the first article to help understand the terminology used in other sections of the issue. Hopefully his very pragmatic approach aids the clinician when reading each of the current review articles that echo the same plea for more controlled clinical evidence based on pharmacokinetic and pharmacodynamic studies.

The order of articles is somewhat phylogenetic, starting with fish analgesia written by Dr Scott Weber. There is tremendous controversy in the fish and amphibian literature questioning if these species are even capable of feeling pain. Dr Weber takes the approach that, whether fish feel pain, are simply fear aversive, or are experiencing nociception to noxious stimuli caused by a variety of factors, it is a veterinary responsibility to help ameliorate this stress or distress as would be done for other livestock, pet, laboratory animal, and wild populations. This article reviews fish neuroanatomical pathways associated with nociception and discusses what is known about behavioral observations in fish, considering the enormous species diversity of this class of animals. This review also summarizes the current analgesic use for the individual fish patient.

No one has contributed more to the amphibian analgesia literature than Dr Craig Stevens, and he was very enthusiastic about writing a review about the clinical application of the available scientific information. He is cautious about making assumptions regarding nociception versus pain and he shares his zoological perspective to help the clinician understand the issues surrounding the use of analgesics in amphibians. Dr Stevens provides the data and the tools for veterinarians to explore the amphibian pain and analgesia literature and challenges us to come to our own evidence-based conclusions.

Reptiles are another class of animals with tremendous species variability affecting neuroanatomy, physiology, and behaviors. Dr Craig Mosley has written several articles on reptile health and in this article provides an excellent review of recent investigations that have aided the veterinarian's decisions to provide analgesia for reptiles. He provides a table of information to assist in the systematic assessment of pain for reptile species. The drug dosage tables provide insightful comments to promote caution and awareness when treating reptiles with analgesics.

The avian analgesia article follows a similar format of reviewing the literature applicable to clinical treatment of avian pain. Pharmacodynamic evaluation of different analgesics in the parrot is my area of research and Dr Michelle Hawkins shares this research interest in birds as well as small mammals. We have joined together in this article to provide the reader with a perspective on current studies and what we know and don't know about interpreting avian behavior and pain relief for birds. Significant contributions have been made studying chickens, waterfowl, and pigeons, and we tried to distill and share the information as it applies to companion birds. The tables in this article are not intended to provide dosages for each of the currently available analgesic therapies, but rather to highlight published studies for the veterinarian to interpret. These research findings can be clinically applied under close observation for analgesic effectiveness in the individual bird.

Using the phylogenetic pattern, the next logical article should be on mammals but fortunately there is significantly more information on this group of zoological companion animals, and small mammals have been divided into separate articles for each of the most common companion species—rodents, rabbits, and ferrets. Dr Linda Barter has a passion for scientific evidence and is very rigorous in her own rabbit analgesia research. Dr Barter and I share some of the same frustrations in trying to adapt analgesimetry methods established in humans to achieve reliable results working with small populations of rabbits or parrots that are adapted to mask painful behaviors. Dr Barter applies her knowledge of domestic animal analgesia to help interpret the current rabbit literature.

The ferret analgesia article was written by a team from the Faculty of Veterinary Medicine at Utrecht University including exotic small mammal clinician Dr Nico Schoemaker, anesthesiologist Dr Joost Uilenreef, and the first author, Dr Hugo van Oostrom, who is an intern in companion animal medicine with his PhD thesis in veterinary analgesia. Despite the ferret being a common laboratory animal species, the paucity of scientific studies on efficacy, pharmacokinetics, pharmacodynamics, and safety of analgesic drugs in the ferret is disappointing. The authors have reviewed the scientific publications as well as the clinical articles on the topic to present how to recognize painful behaviors in ferrets, what analgesic drugs are currently used, and how they can be adopted in a patient-orientated pain management plan for ferrets.

Scientific publications using rodents as models to study pain physiology and analgesia are much more numerous than for other groups of zoological companion animals, and much can be learned from the methods developed for preventing and alleviating pain in animals undergoing research studies. The rodent article is written by authors who are both contributors to advances in rodent analgesia, especially in detection and alleviation of pain and distress in laboratory rodents and the use of behavior-based pain scoring systems. This article reviews advances in pain detection techniques and makes recommendations on available analgesic agents for the treatment of pain.

Tramadol is a relatively new analgesic that is available in an inexpensive, oral form and is not a controlled drug. Tramadol received its own review article because it may be an alternative to other analgesics when treating acute or chronic pain in zoological companion animals. Additionally, tramadol pharmacokinetic and pharmacodynamic studies in zoological species are very current and provide a comparison of the same drug being used to treat various species. This should cause the reader to consider pharmacological principles addressed in the first article by Dr KuKanich. Drs Marcy Souza and Sherry Cox are at the forefront of several tramadol studies in zoological companion animals and provide a review of the drug's mechanism of action and a cross-species review of tramadol use as an analgesic.

Treating pain is not just about giving the right analgesic drug at the right dose for the species in question. The last two articles in this issue were selected to provide information about physical modalities for pain reduction. Physical medicine can be an integral part of recovery from trauma and surgery and typically has fewer adverse effects than conventional medicine. Zoological companion animals are often assumed to be less amenable to physical therapy but they are natural candidates for rehabilitation and benefit with a more rapid and complete recovery. The authors of the rehabilitation and physical medicine article work together to treat birds, reptiles, and exotic small mammals at the University of Colorado with Dr Jessica Rychel and Narda Robinson at the Center for Comparative and Integrative Pain Medicine, and Dr Matthew Johnston as faculty in the Clinical Sciences Department. There are few published studies evaluating physical medicine in these species, and only a few case reports that apply these techniques, but clinical experience adapting the same modalities effectively in domestic animals is an important step toward incorporating techniques such as massage, heat therapy, therapeutic laser, cryotherapy, and exercise.

Acupuncture is one modality of complementary and alternative veterinary medicine presented in the article by Dr Marilyn Koski. Dr Koski is an experienced zoological medicine clinician with advanced training and experience in veterinary acupuncture, so it is a natural process for her to apply acupuncture to the bird, reptile, and small exotic mammal patients. This article is intended to be a primer to understand the principles and applications of acupuncture and is not intended to teach acupuncture techniques to the zoological companion animal veterinarian. Dr Koski provides examples of how the primary clinician can recognize patients that may benefit from acupuncture and how to work with an acupuncturist to address treatment of pain through acupuncture. Many of the zoological companion animal patients are infrequently handled and can be less amenable to calming through tactile or vocal assurance than domesticated animals; however, acupuncture can be used initially in specific calming acupoints to promote relaxation prior to the placement of the remaining needles.

My heartfelt thanks to all of the contributors that have helped to make this issue on analgesia and pain relief for zoological companion animals a very useful tool for investigators, clinicians, animal care-givers, and individuals that want to provide the best possible pain prevention and relief to animals in our care. The message is clear throughout this issue that given the diversity of zoological companion animal species, recognizing painful behaviors and evaluating analgesic efficacy is challenging, since objective measures of behavior associated with pain are difficult to define in nonverbal species, particularly less traditional animal species such as birds, small mammals, reptiles, amphibians, and fish.

Joanne Paul-Murphy, DVM, DACZM
Department of Medicine and Epidemiology
Companion Avian and Exotic Pets
School of Veterinary Medicine
2108 Tupper Hall
One Shields Avenue
University of California
Davis, CA 95616, USA

E-mail address:
paulmurphy@ucdavis.edu

Clinical Interpretation of Pharmacokinetic and Pharmacodynamic Data in Zoologic Companion Animal Species

Butch KuKanich, DVM, PhD, DACVCP

KEYWORDS

- Analgesia • Efficacy • Potency • Half-life • Clearance
- Volume of distribution

The treatment and prevention of pain in zoologic companion animals is difficult because of the lack of data available on the safety and efficacy of drugs. The ideal situation for determining effective drug dosages is with controlled clinical trials, however these are rarely performed in veterinary species because of the high costs of the studies, number of animals needed, and difficulty in working with many of these species. Many dosage recommendations are based on perceived response to therapy, clinical experience, and lack of observable toxicity. However, these extrapolations are difficult to interpret for several reasons. The behavior of companion exotic animals often results in these animals hiding behaviors associated with disease or pain in order to minimize identification as weakened animals by predators or other animals within the herd, pack, or other social group. Therefore signs that are easy to observe in domesticated companion animals, such as lameness in dogs, are difficult to observe in nondomesticated animal species even with a trained and experienced observer.

For example, an animal may seem better after administration of an analgesic, but the pain may not have truly been controlled and the response may be caused by the animal trying to mask the signs in the presence of the observer, by healing of the injury, or by normal variations in pain intensity. The clinical observation in this case would be a perceived improvement after analgesic administration when an improvement did not truly occur. The same treatment is then administered to a similar animal a month later and the same scenario occurs: a perceived improvement when

Funding support: N/A.

College of Veterinary Medicine, Kansas State University, 228 Coles Hall, Manhattan, KS 66506-5802, USA

E-mail address: kukanich@ksu.edu

Vet Clin Exot Anim 14 (2011) 1–20

doi:10.1016/j.cvex.2010.09.006

an improvement did not occur. The clinician now has some confidence that the treatment worked, despite the low number of animals treated, but in reality the analgesic did not work. The clinician then passes the treatment information to another colleague who uses the information with the same perceived improvement when none occurred. The information has then been independently verified and makes its way onto a listserve or by word of mouth at meetings or symposiums to other clinicians and eventually into a formulary. The formulary then undergoes several editions over the years, is referenced by other sources, and the incorrect dosing information becomes dogma. Through nobody's fault, and primarily because of the lack of available objective data, incorrect dosing information can easily become dogma, and this has occurred in veterinary medicine in all species, domesticated and nondomesticated.

The previous scenario emphasizes the importance of objective data and the need for controlled studies in animals. The lack of objective data in zoologic companion animals has numerous causes including the lack of funding, difficulty in handling some animal species, increased animal stress, lack of available animal numbers, the rarity and value of certain species, and the potential for adverse effects. However, without adequate data, therapeutic decisions are difficult to make, especially when treating the large number of animal species, including amphibians, reptiles, birds, and exotic small mammals.

STUDY DESIGNS EVALUATING A THERAPEUTIC AGENT

A logical progression in evaluating a therapeutic agent such as an analgesic would include pharmacokinetic (PK) studies, followed by pharmacodynamic (PD) studies or integrated PK-PD studies, and eventually controlled clinical trials. PK studies evaluate the changes in plasma concentrations over time, the relationship between plasma concentrations and dose, the effects of different routes of administration on the plasma concentrations, and the potential for extrapolating plasma concentrations within a dose range. The effect the drug elicits is not a primary outcome of PK studies. PD studies evaluate the effect produced by the drug after it is administered. PD studies may evaluate a single dose rate or evaluate escalating doses. PK-PD studies integrate changes in drug concentrations versus changes in the effect (ie, whether an increase in dose, or plasma concentration, results in an increase in analgesia). Once a targeted dose is chosen based on PD, or preferably PK-PD, studies, the dose regimen should be evaluated in a controlled clinical trial to confirm that the experimental model accurately predicts the desired effect and lack of adverse effects in clinical patients.

Controlled clinical trials evaluate the test drug in patients clinically affected with an injury or disease, for example, evaluation of a nonsteroidal antiinflammatory drug (NSAID) in ducks with lameness associated with synovitis. In a positive controlled trial, the drug to be tested is compared with a drug known to elicit the desirable effect. For example, a positive controlled trial could include oral meloxicam as the test drug and flunixin as the positive control for the treatment of lameness associated with synovitis. In vivo studies have shown that flunixin inhibits plasma thromboxane for 6 to 12 hours in mallard ducks.[1] Some assumptions in positive controlled trials include that previous studies have shown that the positive control is effective in the species to be tested, the positive control is effective at the administered dosage, the duration of effect of the positive control has been determined, and the positive control is effective for the specified disease. However, there are few clinical studies in nondomestic species that meet these assumptions. Limitations of the lame duck example are: flunixin has not been shown to produce analgesic effects in ducks or in ducks with synovitis; the dose of flunixin was determined in an experimental model (inhibition of plasma thromboxane) and may not extrapolate to analgesia for synovitis; the dose of flunixin was determined in healthy animals, not in animals with an inflammatory condition; and the test dose of oral meloxicam is undetermined, so the oral bioavailability may be lower than estimated and the lack of a response caused by the dose being too low, not lack of efficacy.

A placebo-controlled clinical study evaluates the test drug against a treatment that is known not to elicit a clinical effect. For example, tramadol is administered in capsules to 1 group of rabbits, a second group of rabbits is administered capsules containing lactose, and both groups are evaluated for improvement in pain from naturally occurring osteoarthritis. A criticism of placebo-controlled trials is that 1 group of animals is not receiving an analgesic. However, it is questionable where the greater harm is: a placebo-controlled study in 20 animals (half of which receive the analgesic to be tested), or conducting a clinical trial with a positive control that has not been shown to be more effective than a placebo. The problem with an unvalidated positive control is the interpretation when no significant difference is seen between the unvalidated positive control and test drug groups. No significant difference is just as likely to mean that neither drug elicited an effect as that both drugs elicited an effect. If neither drug elicited an effect, than the net result may be hundreds, thousands, or potentially millions of animals receiving an ineffective drug, compared with 10/20 animals receiving a placebo.

The ideal controlled clinical study would also involve randomization of test groups and all investigators directly involved in the study being blinded to the administered treatments. Randomization avoids bias in selecting animals to receive the test drug and the control drug. For example, a ferret may be enrolled in a placebo-controlled clinical trial evaluating an NSAID for the control of osteoarthritis. The ferret is 3/4 lame, therefore the investigators put the ferret in the NSAID treatment group, whereas a ferret with a 1/4 lameness is put into the placebo group. The biased assignment of animals into the test groups could affect the results of the trial by placing animals with the most severe lameness in the NSAID-treated group. However, the lameness in the animals in the treatment group may have been so severe that it would be nonresponsive to NSAIDs. The interpretation could erroneously be made that the NSAID was ineffective, but the severity of the arthritis was the primary reason for the poor efficacy. Conversely, assignment of less severely affected animals to the placebo group could bias the results in favor of the NSAID-treated group because of the potential magnitude of change being more limited in the placebo group. For example, the initial average lameness in the placebo group may have only been 1/4 at the beginning of the study, with the final lameness graded at 0.5/4, a change in magnitude of 0.5 units. The treated group may have had an initial lameness score of 2.5/4 lame, which improved to 1.5/4 lame, resulting in a greater magnitude of change (1 unit) and potentially erroneously interpreting the results as the NSAID having a greater effect than placebo, when the real effect was normal variation in the disease. An alternative way of assessing these data would be a 50% improvement (0.5 final lameness/1.0 initial lameness) in the placebo group compared with a 40% improvement (1.5 final lameness/2.5 initial lameness) in the NSAID-treated group, which could bias the results in favor of the placebo because of bias in the assignment to treatment groups. In addition, the blinding of the investigators to the treatments is intended to minimize either intentional or unintentional bias when evaluating the pivotal parameter in the study. For example, in evaluating the effects of an NSAID on lameness in ferrets, the investigator may subconsciously think the NSAID-treated group must be doing better than the placebo group, and as a result the scores for lameness are more improved in the treatment group compared with the placebo group.

Another important component of clinical trials is the detection of adverse effects that may not have been previously reported. Because the treatment is administered to clinical patients, instead of young healthy patients, the rate of adverse effects in the clinical trial is often greater. This information is extremely valuable because it may provide guidelines for adverse effect monitoring, patient selection, potential for drug-drug interactions, and recommendations for clinical chemistry/complete blood count monitoring in addition to drug efficacy. A good example of reported adverse effects in clinical trials involved the approval of meloxicam in domestic cats. During the positive controlled (butorphanol), randomized, and blinded clinical trial, 8.3% of cats experienced increases in the blood urea nitrogen (BUN) in the meloxicam-treated group, but none of the cats experienced BUN changes in the butorphanol-treated groups.[2] The increased BUN suggested that the NSAID caused some adverse effects in the kidneys of cats, which was later confirmed once the drug was released and adverse effects were reported to the US Food and Drug Administration.

Ideally, drug studies in zoologic companion animals would also involve toxicology studies. However, the rarity and value of many of these animals preclude toxicology studies. Valuable information is gained from toxicology studies, including potential adverse effects, range of dosages administered with no toxic effect levels, breed- or species-specific differences in toxicology, and a relative confidence in the safety of the drug. As an example, toxicology studies in domestic cats indicated that the toxic doses of acetaminophen overlap therapeutic doses, therefore no dose of acetaminophen in domestic cats is safe and effective.[3]

PKs
Primer on PKs

PKs is the use of mathematical models to predict plasma drug concentrations in the body. The primary PK parameters are the terminal half-life ($T_{1/2}$), clearance (Cl), and volume of distribution (V_d). The maximum plasma concentration (CMAX), time to CMAX (TMAX) and area under the curve (AUC) are also useful PK parameters.

The $T_{1/2}$ is the time it takes for the plasma concentration to decrease by 50%.[4] It is often incorrectly stated as the amount of time it takes to eliminate half of the drug. Decreases in plasma drug concentrations are not always caused by drug elimination, but could be caused by drug redistribution from the plasma to other tissues. The $T_{1/2}$ is a useful parameter because it allows the estimation for decreases in plasma drug concentrations, time needed for drug to reach steady state, and the ratio of peaks and troughs.

By definition, for every $T_{1/2}$ the plasma concentration decreases by 50% (**Table 1**), therefore some predictions of changes in plasma concentrations can be made if the $T_{1/2}$ is known. After $3 \times T_{1/2}$, the plasma concentration will have decreased by $\sim 88\%$; after $5 \times T_{1/2}$, the plasma concentration will have decreased by $\sim 97\%$; and by $7 \times T_{1/2}$, the plasma concentration will have decreased by $\sim 99\%$. This estimate can be useful in determining washout periods, treatment of certain intoxications, and sometimes durations of drug effect. The $T_{1/2}$ also predicts the time it takes for a drug to reach steady state drug concentrations if given by multiple doses or by a constant rate infusion. The time to steady state can be predicted in a similar manner to predictions for decreases plasma concentration; that is, $\sim 88\%$ of steady state will be achieved in $3 \times T_{1/2}$, 97% of steady state will be achieved in $5 \times T_{1/2}$, and 99% of steady state will be achieved in $7 \times T_{1/2}$. As an example, a drug that has a $T_{1/2}$ of 24 hours will reach 88% of steady state in 72 hours ($3 \times T_{1/2}$), 97% of steady state in 120 hours ($5 \times T_{1/2}$), and 99% of steady state plasma concentrations in 168 hours

Table 1
The percentage decrease in plasma drug concentration as a function of the number of half-lives

Number of Half-lives	Percentage of Initial Drug Concentration Remaining in Plasma	Percentage of Drug Concentration Decrease in Plasma
0	100	0
1	50	50
2	25	75
3	12.5	87.5
4	6.25	93.75
5	3.125	96.875
6	1.5625	98.4375
7	0.78125	99.21875
8	0.390625	99.609375
9	0.1953125	99.8046875
10	0.09765625	99.9023438

$(7 \times T_{1/2})$. The $T_{1/2}$, along with the dosing interval, can also be used to predict the fluctuations in peak and trough plasma drug concentrations. If the $T_{1/2}$ is much shorter than the dosing interval, most of the drug will be eliminated before the next dose, resulting in a large fluctuation between peak and trough concentrations. A drug with a short $T_{1/2}$ (1 hour, for example) administered every 8 hours will have large fluctuations in peak and trough concentrations because there will be a large decrease in plasma concentrations before the next dose (>99%; **Fig. 1A**). Conversely, if the $T_{1/2}$ is much greater than the dosing interval, there will be less fluctuation in plasma concentrations as minimal decreases occur before the next dose is administered, and the result is minimal fluctuation between peak and trough concentrations. A drug with a 48-hour $T_{1/2}$ administered once daily (every 24 hours) will have slight decreases in plasma concentrations before the next dose ($\sim$25%; see **Fig. 1B**).

The apparent V_d is the apparent volume that a drug dilutes into after administration. The V_d is not necessarily a true physiologic volume. The V_d is species specific and formulation specific, and even age specific, therefore extrapolations must be made cautiously (see later discussion). The V_d is readily calculated with the following equation if the dose and drug concentration after intravenous (IV) administration are known: V_d = dose/concentration. The primary usefulness of the V_d is to calculate a loading dose to immediately achieve desired concentrations by rearranging the equation to: dose = $V_d \times$concentration.

A loading dose is most critical when immediate effects are wanted from a drug with a long $T_{1/2}$ because of the prolonged time to steady state (see earlier discussion). As an example, phenobarbital has a V_d in dogs of 700 mL kg^{-1} and 20 μg mL^{-1} is within the reported range of therapeutic plasma concentrations. Therefore the dose can be calculated by multiplying the V_d (700 mL kg^{-1} in this example) by the targeted concentration (20 μg mL^{-1}): (700 mL kg^{-1})$\times$(20 μg mL^{-1}) = 14,000 μg kg^{-1} = 14 mg kg^{-1}. Another use of the V_d is to estimate a dose in a species for which the drug has not yet been examined. The V_d can be estimated through allometric analysis (see later discussion), but there are numerous limitations to this approach, including the lack of a dosing interval.

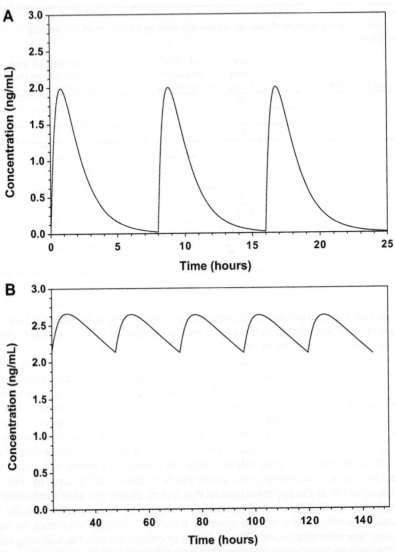

Fig. 1. The peak and trough ratio can be estimated based on the $T_{1/2}$ and dosing interval. (A) The $T_{1/2}$ (1 hour) is much shorter than the dosing interval (every 8 hours), in this case resulting in a large fluctuation (100-fold) in the peak and trough concentrations. (B) The $T_{1/2}$ (48 hours) is much greater than the dosing interval (every 24 hours) resulting in minimal fluctuation (0.25-fold) in the peak and trough concentrations.

The plasma Cl of a drug is the volume of the body for which the drug distributes cleared of the drug per unit time (ie, the volume of the V_d cleared per unit time). Plasma Cl is the sum of all mechanisms of drug elimination, including renal (glomerular filtration, tubular secretion, and renal metabolism), hepatic (metabolism and biliary secretion), and other clearance mechanism such as plasma esterases, monoamine oxidases, and splenic and intestinal metabolism. The usefulness of the clearance parameter is in calculating a constant rate infusion or average plasma drug concentrations using the equation: dose rate = Cl×steady state drug concentration. As an example, the clearance of morphine in llamas[5] is 27.3 mL min^{-1} kg^{-1} and a plasma drug concentration of 20 ng mL^{-1} is desired, then the dose can be calculated as follows: dose rate = (27.3 mL min^{-1} kg^{-1})×(20 ng mL^{-1}) = 546 ng min^{-1} kg^{-1} = 32,760 ng h^{-1} kg^{-1} = 0.03276 mg h^{-1} kg^{-1}.

The AUC is the calculated area under the curve of plasma concentration versus time (**Fig. 2**). The AUC is a measure of cumulative drug exposure and is related to the dose administered, plasma drug concentrations, and the duration of time the plasma drug concentrations persist. The AUC is proportional to the dose for most drugs; for example, doubling the dose results in a doubling of the AUC. In addition, because the AUC is dependent on the time the drug concentrations persist in the plasma, increases in half-life caused by decreased drug elimination result in increases in the AUC. The efficacy of some drugs is best correlated with the AUC. As an example aspirin efficacy in humans for postoperative dental pain is well correlated with the plasma AUC; the higher the aspirin AUC the better the pain control.[6] The correlation for aspirin analgesia was better for the AUC than the CMAX. The toxicities of some drugs have also been correlated with the AUC; for example, the antiplatelet effects of aspirin are correlated with the AUC of aspirin in humans, therefore the prevalence of excessive bleeding is expected to increase as the aspirin AUC increases.[7] The AUC is also a pivotal parameter in the determination of drug bioavailability, with the AUC from the extravascular route divided by the AUC of IV administration. The AUC is also a pivotal parameter in the determination of drug bioequivalence when comparing different drug formulations (ie, a brand name drug versus a generic drug).

The CMAX is the maximum drug concentration after extravascular administration (see **Fig. 2**). The CMAX is typically proportional to the dose, so, for example, doubling the dose typically results in a doubling of the CMAX, whereas decreasing the dose by 50% decreases the CMAX by 50%. The CMAX has been correlated with toxicity for

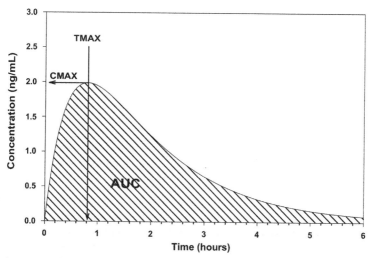

Fig. 2. The PK parameters: maximum plasma concentration (CMAX = 2 ng mL^{-1}), time to maximum plasma concentration (TMAX = 0.8 hours) and AUC (5 ng h mL^{-1}), represented as the hashed area.

many different drugs and efficacy for some drugs. For example, the toxicity of sevo-flurane is related to achieving high concentrations, which cause respiratory depression and death.[8] The CMAX is the second pivotal parameter for drug bioequivalence when comparing 2 different drug formulations (ie, a brand name drug vs a generic drug). The TMAX is the time of the CMAX and is typically constant for a drug formulation regardless of dose, so a doubling of the dose results in no change in the TMAX. To determine the peak drug concentration, the CMAX, for therapeutic drug monitoring, the plasma sample will be obtained at the TMAX.

Analytical Methods for PK Studies

The method of drug analysis can greatly affect the PK parameters. Numerous different methodologies are available, but direct comparisons cannot be made when different methods of analysis are used. Mass spectrometry methods tend to be highly sensitive, measuring very low concentrations, and are highly specific, with minimal cross-reactivity with metabolites or endogenous substances and xenobiotics. Mass spectrometry is often considered the analytical method of choice, but it is among the most expensive methods available and requires expensive equipment and substantial training to use. Mass spectrometry is typically coupled to gas chromatography or high-pressure liquid chromatography (HPLC).

HPLC and gas chromatography (GC) tend to have moderate sensitivity and low to moderate specificity. Most compounds can be accurately and precisely quantified with HPLC and GC, but high-potency drugs (low drug concentrations to achieve an effect), or drugs that are extensively metabolized to numerous metabolites, can be difficult to accurately and precisely measure by HPLC and GC. HPLC and GC costs are moderate, as is the technical expertise required to use these systems.

Immunoassays, including radioimmunoassay (RIAs), enzyme linked immunoassays (ELISAs), and fluorescence polarization immunoassays (FPIAs) are usually adequately sensitive, but the specificity is variable. Immunoassays may cross-react with metabolites or other drugs, can overestimate drug concentrations, and are typically considered to have less specificity than the other methods of analysis. However, drugs that are minimally metabolized can be accurately and precisely measured by immunoassays. There are some immunoassays that are highly specific for some drugs that are metabolized, but many of these have not been validated in animals in which the metabolic pathways and drug metabolites have not been identified. Immunoassays tend to have lower costs than other analytical methods and tend to be technically less difficult to run.

Direct comparisons of PK results using different analytical methods can be difficult because of differences in sensitivity and specificity in analytical methods (see later discussion). Ideally, a full method validation for each species being evaluated should be included for each drug analyzed and should be performed in the laboratory performing the drug analysis in order to assure the most accurate results, including assessment of cross-reactivity of metabolites, xenobiotics, and endogenous substances.

PK studies

The purpose of PK studies is to describe the changes in plasma concentrations over time, the relationship between plasma concentrations and dose, the effects of different routes of administration on the plasma concentrations, and the potential for extrapolating plasma concentrations within a dose range. The end goal is often to correlate physiologic processes with the PK model and use the data to make predictions of when parameters may change, as in renal or hepatic disease or species difference.[9] PK studies most often involve determining the drug concentration in plasma or serum, because these are typically the easiest and most readily obtained samples. Plasma and serum samples also have been most often correlated with a clinical effect, despite the blood, plasma, or serum rarely being the location of the body where the drug has its effect. Other areas of the body are occasionally sampled, such as synovial fluid, cerebrospinal fluid (CSF), whole tissues, urine, and feces, but, because of difficulties in collection from many of these areas or because of urine and feces contain the concentrations of the drugs after they have been metabolized and eliminated from the body, they are less frequently used in PK studies.

PK Study Design

There are numerous different methods of PK study design. The most common method is termed the standard 2-stage (STS) method. The basic design of an STS is to administer a drug to a small homogenous group of animals, collect many samples from individual animals, analyze each sample independently, calculate the PK parameters for each animal individually, and report the descriptive statistics of the PK parameters, such as mean, median, and range. The advantages of an STS include a robust estimate of the average PK parameters in the homogenous population; a small number of animals is included, which subsequently minimizes the facilities needed; relative ease of sample collection in some animals; potential for training the animals for handling and sampling; and the short time in which the study can be completed. However, numerous limitations of the STS method are also present. Small numbers of homogenous animals are studied, which limits the direct application of the data to that well-defined group of animals. Many variables may not be accounted for in an STS study such as disease and concurrent medications, the effects of age, the variability within the entire animal population, breed- and sometimes gender-specific differences, outliers are often not identified, the potential stress from obtaining multiple samples from an individual animal, and volume depletion from repeated sampling from small animals. A recent study examined the PK of oral tramadol in rabbits using an STS method.[10] Six healthy, sexually intact New Zealand White female rabbits, weighing 3.8 ($\pm$ 0.38) kg were administered oral tramadol. Although robust parameters were reported, it is unclear whether these parameters are applicable to animals with underlying disease, perioperative patients, young or geriatric animals, and animals administered concurrent drugs, among other variables.

Naïve Average and Naïve Pooled Analysis

Naïve averaged or naïve pooled PK studies are often used in captive wild animals, zoologic companion animals, small animals, or animals in which samples are difficult to obtain. Fewer samples are collected from each individual, precluding the calculation of individual PK parameters. Instead the individual samples are analyzed, the average concentration at each time point is determined, and the PK model is fitted to the average concentrations. One of the disadvantages to this approach is that the variability within the PK parameters cannot be determined. In addition, bimodal distributions may not be identified using this model. Many of the disadvantages of the STS method still occur using naïve average analysis if homogenous animal populations are used. A variant of the naïve average analysis is the naïve pooled analysis. Naïve pooled analysis involves using all samples collected and fitting a model to all of the samples without first calculating the average plasma concentrations at each time point. An advantage of the naïve pooled analysis is that the time points do not have to be as precise because the average concentration for each time point is not calculated. For example, naïve average analysis of buprenorphine in mice collected samples from 4 different animals at each of the following times: 5, 15, and 30 minutes and 1, 2, 3, 5,

7, 9, 12, 18, and 24 hours after drug administration for a total of 48 animals.[11] The average concentrations at each time point were then calculated and the PK model fitted to the average concentrations. Problems can occur in naïve averaged analysis if an animal is difficult to bleed, resulting in the sample being collected 15 minutes late, or if the sample is missed entirely. Naïve pooled analysis is less affected by late time points or time points in which samples are missed, assuming the final data are appropriately distributed throughout the sampling period to avoid bias. Extensive studies examining whether either the naïve averaged or naïve pooled method are more robust are lacking. A study evaluating the PK of oral marbofloxacin in harbor seals compared these methods of analysis and suggested that the primary PK parameters were similar regardless of the method used.[12]

Population PK Analysis

Population PK modeling, also referred to as mixed effects modeling, is a complex modeling scheme in which a large number of subjects are included in the study (hundreds to thousands are included in human studies), and a very limited number of samples obtained from each individual. Population PK analysis has some advantages but, because of the large number of subjects required, it is beyond the scope of this article. A thorough review of population PK is published elsewhere.[13]

Allometric Analysis

Allometric analysis is used to estimate the PK parameters of a drug in a species for which data are not available, but data are available in numerous other species. Allometric analysis is a mathematical approach for estimating PK parameters before administering a drug to an animal. The principle of allometric scaling is that major physiologic processes are related to body weight raised to some power.[14] The basic allometric equation is $Y = a \times weight^b$, where Y is the PK parameter to be estimated, a is the allometric coefficient, weight is the weight of the animal, and b is the allometric exponent. The PK parameters typically estimated are the clearance and V_d. $T_{1/2}$ is occasionally estimated, but it is a function of the clearance and V_d ($T_{1/2} = 0.693 \times V_d/Cl$) and therefore it does not have to be estimated. In addition, $T_{1/2}$ tends to extrapolate poorly.

Allometric analysis is an estimator and not a calculator of PK parameters. There are numerous reports detailing the potential inaccuracy of allometric scaling,[15,16] but it has proven useful for some drugs and species.[15,17,18] One of the considerations for allometric analysis is the extrapolation of data only within the range of data available. For example, data on the PK of intravenous buprenorphine are available from mice (0.027 kg) to horses (525 kg) (**Table 2**), therefore extrapolation to an elephant weighing 2000 kg is inappropriate because it is outside the weight range and may not be accurate. Extrapolation between different classes of animals, such as birds, mammals, reptiles, and amphibians is also likely inaccurate because of the vast differences in physiology of these species. Species-specific differences in metabolism must also be considered; for example, cats are poor at glucuronide conjugate formation, dogs are poor at acetyl conjugation, some dogs are deficient in p-glycoprotein drug transporters.[19,20] Differences in metabolism have been documented in rats, primarily because of their use as laboratory animals. Sprague-Dawley rats from 2 different sources had significantly different metabolism of morphine; rats from Denmark had significantly faster metabolism of morphine compared with rats from Sweden, and subsequently the rats from Denmark had significantly less analgesia when administered the same morphine dose.[21] It is expected that differences in other zoologic companion animals are also present, but not yet documented.

Table 2
PK parameters of intravenous buprenorphine in a variety of species; predicted parameters based on allometric analysis and accuracy of the predicted parameters

PK Parameter		Mice[11]	Rats[46]	Dogs[47]	Goats[48]	Humans[49]	Alpacas[50]	Horses[51]
$T_{1/2}$ (h)	Actual	2.9	5.28	9.0	1.1	3.21	2.3	7.14
	Predicted	2.87	2.87	2.87	2.87	2.87	2.87	2.87
	Accuracy (%)	99	54	32	261	89	125	40
Cl (mL min^{-1})	Actual	1.94	8.1	336	3188	1281	4274.66	4147.5
	Predicted	1.99	9.12	299.63	695.47	1089.45	1215.04	5483.58
	Accuracy (%)	103	113	89	22	85	28	132
V_d at steady state (L)	Actual	0.176	1.507	133	201.6	334.6	569.42	1785
	Predicted	0.211	1.254	75.116	201.535	341.058	387.584	2267.091
	Accuracy (%)	120	83	56	100	102	68	127
Weight (kg)		0.027	0.18	14	40	70	80.2	525

To perform an allometric analysis, data from previous PK studies are collected from a variety of species with a large range in weights. Each parameter ($T_{1/2}$, Cl, V_d) is estimated independently in allometric analysis. The logarithm of the absolute value of the parameter (mL min^{-1} not mL min^{-1} kg^{-1}) is plotted against the logarithm of body weight (**Figs. 3–5**). A regression analysis is then performed for each parameter fitting the allometric equation. A weighting factor can be added to better fit the equation to the data, especially for animals with lower body weights. As an example, an allometric analysis of buprenorphine is included (see **Figs. 3–5**, see **Table 2**). Data from animals in which PK studies were performed and drug concentrations were determined using mass spectrometry methods were included in the allometric analysis. Other methods of analysis are not included because of potential bias in the data (see earlier discussion).

The allometric analysis of buprenorphine yielded variable results. As expected, the half-life scaled poorly (see **Fig. 3**). The scaling of the clearance was moderate, with an R^2 of 0.7688, which is a reasonable coefficient of determination (**Fig. 4**). However, examining the allometric predicted results with the published values shows one of the weaknesses of this method of prediction. The predicted values for goats and alpacas are markedly lower than observed, indicating that allometric analysis is not a good estimator for every species, but the other species were within 32% of the actual values. As stated previously, the clearance is a useful parameter in estimating the average plasma concentration or steady state concentration in a multiple dose protocol or continuous infusion. The V_d for buprenorphine scaled the best, with an R^2 of 0.9249 (**Fig. 5**). Even with a high coefficient of determination, the predicted value for dogs was only 56% of the actual value, indicating that it is not an accurate estimator for all species despite a high correlation. The V_d, as discussed earlier, is useful for estimating the initial plasma concentrations for drug administration and can be used to determine an initial dose.

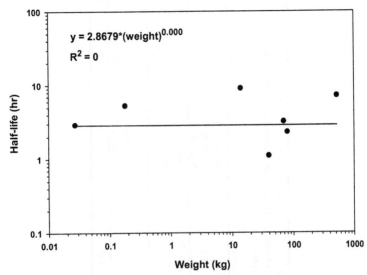

Fig. 3. Allometric analysis of the elimination half-life of buprenorphine. See **Table 2** for species and PK parameters used in the allometric analysis. A weighting factor of 1/y was used for the analysis.

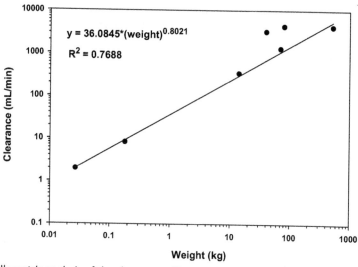

Fig. 4. Allometric analysis of the clearance of buprenorphine. See **Table 2** for species and PK parameters used in the allometric analysis. A weighting factor of $1/(y^2)$ was used for the analysis.

Application of allometric scaling

Allometric scaling could be used for determining a dose in a clinical patient, but is often applied before the design of a PK study. For example, what buprenorphine dose should be administered IV to assess the PK of buprenorphine in 400 g (0.4 kg) hedgehogs? The V_d can be estimated with the allometric equation from **Fig. 5**: $V_d = 6.2844 \times 0.4^{0.9401} = 2.656$ L or 6.639 L kg^{-1}. If an initial plasma concentration of 5 ng mL^{-1} is desired, the dose can be calculated using the equation: Dose = $V_d \times$

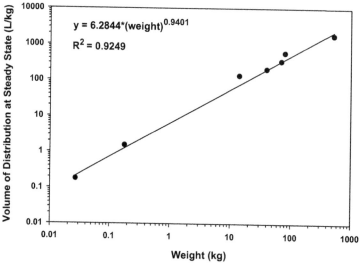

Fig. 5. Allometric analysis of the V_d at steady state of buprenorphine. See **Table 2** for species and PK parameters used in the allometric analysis. A weighting factor of $1/(y^2)$ was used for the analysis.

concentration = (6.639 L kg^{-1}) × (5 ng*mL^{-1}) = (6.639 L kg^{-1}) × (5000 ng L^{-1}) = 33,195 ng kg^{-1} = 33.2 µg kg^{-1} = 0.033 mg kg^{-1}. Because of the variable elimination reported for buprenorphine, a sampling strategy would likely include collecting samples to 24 hours.

PD AND PK-PD STUDIES
PD Studies Overview

The purpose of PD studies is to determine the effects a drug elicits after administration. PD studies can use either healthy animals, if an appropriate model is available, or clinically affected animals. PD studies are critical, especially with the wide variety of species that need to be treated in veterinary medicine and previously described species-specific differences. Extrapolations are often made from plasma drug concentrations or dosages in other species, but it is unknown whether the species to be treated will respond similarly to similar drug concentrations.

Efficacy and potency

Efficacy and potency are PD terms that are often incorrectly used interchangeably. Efficacy describes the maximum effect elicited when a drug is administered at increasing doses. In contrast, potency describes the dose or concentration required to elicit an effect. Drugs with greater potency are not necessarily more effective than drugs with less potency, but drugs with greater potency require lower concentrations (doses) than drugs with a lower potency. Opioids provide an example of comparisons of efficacy and potency. Fentanyl, morphine, and buprenorphine are opioids used in rats. Morphine and fentanyl are µ opioid agonists that produce the maximum analgesic effect possible for opioids in rats before loss of consciousness, whereas buprenorphine is a partial µ agonist producing a submaximum analgesic effect in rats.[22] Therefore, in rats, morphine and fentanyl have similar efficacy and buprenorphine has lower efficacy (**Fig. 6**). The rank order of efficacy is buprenorphine < morphine = fentanyl in rats. In contrast, the potency of fentanyl is greater than morphine and buprenorphine has similar potency to fentanyl. The rank order of potency is morphine < buprenorphine = fentanyl in rats. Potency and efficacy are independent parameters, and the efficacy and potency may differ depending on the species investigated.

PD and PK-PD models

PD analgesic models are difficult to conduct in nonrodent animals. A variety of models are accepted in rodents, but their use in other animal species is not always applicable or appropriate. An extensive review of analgesic modeling has been previously published.[23] Four basic types of noxious stimuli models are used in animals, including electrical stimulation, temperature stimulation (heat and cold), mechanical stimulation, and chemical stimulation. Each type of model has advantages and disadvantages and are addressed briefly in this article; however, extensive detail is available elsewhere.[23]

Electrical stimulation induces nerve depolarization, which is not specific to nociceptors, therefore, even with an effective analgesic, neurons other than those associated with pain, such as heat and cold, autonomic functions, muscle, and touch will be activated, which makes interpretation difficult. Electrical stimulation may not mimic clinical pain syndromes, which may lead to inappropriate conclusions.[23] Electrical stimulation models have been used by various groups to show opioid induced analgesia in birds,[24-26] and is used in humans.[23]

Models using temperature stimulation are most often performed using heat stimuli, but cold can also be effective. Use of temperature stimulation is also not specific for

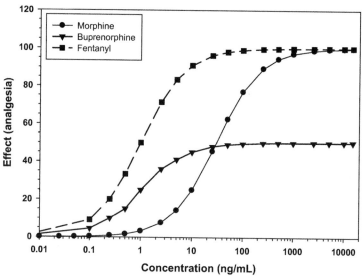

Fig. 6. Comparison of theoretic PDs of the opioids morphine, buprenorphine, and fentanyl in rats. The concentration of the drug is represented on the x-axis (log scale) and the analgesic effect is represented on the y-axis. As the concentration of each drug is increased, an increase in the analgesic effect occurs until it reaches a plateau after which further increases in drug concentrations do not result in an increase in effect. In this example, the rank of efficacy is buprenorphine < morphine = fentanyl and the rank of potency is morphine < buprenorphine = fentanyl.

nociceptors because both cold or heat receptors can be activated. In addition, the use of thermodes also provides a mechanical stimulation that may affect the results. A carbon dioxide laser system may be most effective, but high cost, technical expertise, and persistent pain and damage may occur.[23] Thermal nociception models have been used in nondomestic animals including rodents, birds, snakes, turtles, and crocodiles,[22,26–30] and are used in humans.[23]

Mechanical models produce stimulation through force on a specific part of the body. The von Frey model is the classic example of a mechanical stimulation model in which a filament or rigid plastic tip is applied with increasing force until nociception occurs. A disadvantage of this model is that it activates pressure sensory (touch) nerves in addition to nociceptors. Mechanical stimulation models primarily activate the fast-response, Aδ fibers nociceptors, which are associated with sharp, well-discerned pain, whereas clinical pain occurs primarily from the slow-response, c-fibers, which produce dull, aching, poorly localized pain.[23] Mechanical models are most commonly used in rodents,[31,32] but have been used in other veterinary species, and are used in humans.[23]

Chemical models of nociception inject a chemical that causes pain (an algesic) and some of the chemical algesics also cause inflammation. Chemical stimulation most closely mimics clinical pain.[23] However, chemical algesics also have limitations. The nociception increases to a peak and then decreases, therefore the stimulus is not constant throughout the experiment. The stimulus typically cannot be stopped once started. Many chemical models also produce concurrent inflammation, therefore direct comparisons of analgesics with antiinflammatory effects (ie, nonsteroidal antiinflammatory drugs) with analgesics without substantial antiinflammatory effects (ie, opioids) result in the assessment of different effects (analgesia and antiinflammatory effects vs analgesic effects). Chemical stimulation models have been used in birds to evaluate the efficacy of analgesics,[33,34] and are used in humans.[23]

PD and PK-PD modeling

The potency and efficacy of a drug may be determined in different ways. The 2 primary methods are dose-response and concentration-response methods. Concentration-response methods determine the drug concentration (typically plasma) and correlate it with the analgesic response. Disadvantages of concentration-response studies are the need to obtain multiple plasma samples, the typically high cost of drug analysis, and that the act of obtaining the samples can also interfere with the analysis of the analgesic effect. However, concentration-response analysis provides data that are more readily extrapolated to other routes of administration, different formulations, and provide better intra- and interanimal comparisons of potency and efficacy.

A drawback of using a concentration-response PD study is that plasma drug concentrations are typically being measured, but the effect of the drug typically occurs in a different anatomic location. A lag from the maximum plasma concentration to the maximum drug effect and a lag from the time when drug concentrations begin to decrease and the loss of analgesic effect often occurs, a phenomenon termed hysteresis. However, a variety of PD models are available to account for hysteresis and this modeling strategy has been used to describe the PD of morphine in veterinary species.[35]

Some investigators have proposed measuring CSF as a better method of determining the concentration-effect relationship of opioids. However, the CSF is not the effect compartment, CSF drug concentrations are not directly related to the drug effects in many cases, and CSF samples are more difficult to obtain than plasma.[36,37] Although CSF concentrations may represent a component of the lag that occurs from drug diffusing from the plasma to the central nervous system (CNS), the drug still must diffuse from the CSF into the parenchyma of the CNS and bind to opioid receptors within the brain and spinal cord to elicit the effect.[37] Obtaining CSF is more difficult and invasive than obtaining plasma, and has minimal benefits to PK-PD modeling.

Dose-response methods administer increasing doses of the drug and measure the response to the different doses. Limitations of dose-response studies are the lack of correlation with the concentrations and PK of the drug. Therefore, differences in PK parameters (eg, bioavailability, V_d, $T_{1/2}$) may result in inaccurate conclusions as to the drug's efficacy and potency if only dose-response relationships are evaluated. For example, morphine has an oral bioavailability of 5% in dogs[38] compared with 40% in humans,[39] so comparing a dose-response relationship would result in inaccurately stating that morphine is 8 times more potent in humans than in dogs. However, if a concentration-response study is performed, the effect of morphine in relation to plasma drug concentrations is similar in both species, indicating equal potencies. Therefore, the true differences of oral morphine in dogs and humans are PK differences, not PD differences. Another limitation of dose-response studies is that incorrect conclusions about drug efficacy could be made if a single dose, or small a range of doses, is administered. Again, the example of oral morphine in dogs would have resulted in the conclusion that morphine is ineffective in dogs if only examined at a dose range from 0.1 to 2.2 mg kg^{-1} orally, because of the poor oral bioavailability, but in reality morphine is highly effective in dogs if adequate plasma concentrations are achieved.[35,40,41] A similar situation has been documented in rats, in which Sprague-Dawley rats from 2 different sources had significantly different PK, which, if unaccounted for, would have led to the erroneous conclusion that morphine was an effective analgesic in rats from once source but not the other.[21] Therefore, lack of effectiveness for drugs in which large ranges of doses or no PK information is available has to be interpreted cautiously. The lack of effect may be caused by a true lack of efficacy or inappropriate doses being assessed.

PK-PD modeling is a modeling strategy that incorporates both the PK and PD components simultaneously. An advantage of PK-PD modeling is that changes in the PK of the drug (ie, decreased elimination from hepatic or renal failure, extended release formulations, infusions vs bolus administration, and so forth) can be incorporated into the model and predictions of the changes in drug effect can be made. These predictions are based on the changes in the PK, with the assumption that the activity of the drug itself will remain unchanged. Some veterinary studies have included PK-PD models, but these are less frequently performed than either PK or PD studies.[35]

True PD studies in zoologic companion animals are not routinely performed for numerous reasons including cost, animal availability, difficulty in working with some of the species, and humane reasons. Some exceptions are the species that are also considered laboratory animals, such as mice and rats. Therefore, extrapolations of effective concentrations between species are often made. For example, the effective plasma concentration (EC50) of morphine in male humans and female humans has been reported to be 21 and 11 ng mL^{-1}, respectively.[42] The EC50 of morphine in dogs has been reported to be 23.9 and 29.5 for multiple IV doses and IV infusion, respectively.[40] A separate study found excellent correlations between the effective plasma concentrations of morphine and 6 other opioids (R^2 = 0.949) between mice and humans,[43] suggesting that extrapolations between some species may be appropriate. However, the reported effective concentration of morphine in llamas was 85 ng mL^{-1}, which is substantially higher than that reported in humans, dogs, and mice, but the studies all used different analgesic models, which may also affect the extrapolation of effective drug concentrations.[5]

An example of species-specific differences in PD occurs with xylazine in dogs, cattle, and horses, despite similar PK parameters and near-dose proportional plasma concentrations.[44,45] The effective dose of xylazine is approximately 1.1 mg kg^{-1} IV in dogs, 1.1 mg kg^{-1} IV in horses, and 0.1 mg kg^{-1} IV in ruminants.[45] The plasma concentrations are approximately dose proportional between species, in which cattle have the lowest xylazine plasma concentrations and dogs have the highest plasma concentrations after administration of an effective dose, suggesting a true difference in the sensitivity of each species to the sedative effects of xylazine.[44] Similarly, there seem to be differences to the sensitivity of xylazine even within Cervidae, with fallow deer (*Dama dama*) requiring 1.1 to 2.2 mg kg^{-1} intramuscular (IM), whereas white-tailed deer (*Odocoileus virginianus*) require 0.5 to 1.1 mg kg^{-1}, and elk (*Cervus canadensis*) require a dose of 0.1 to 0.25 mg kg^{-1} IM.[45] However, the PK of xylazine are not available between the different species of Cervidae, therefore allometric differences or differences in other PK parameters, such as bioavailability, V_d, and $T_{1/2}$, cannot be ruled out in these species.

SUMMARY

PK studies are useful for determining the effect of dose on plasma concentrations, duration of detectable plasma concentrations, and reasonable routes of administration. However, species-specific differences in a drug's PK can occur, resulting in poor extrapolation between animal species. PK data can also be affected within a species by physiologic factors such as concurrent disease or organ impairment, or by drug-drug interactions. PK data are also influenced by the analytical method used to determine plasma drug concentrations, study design, and method of PK analysis. Therefore, different studies may not be comparable. PK studies and data do not in themselves determine effective drug dosages, but are a vital component for determining the potential for the use of a drug within an animal species.

PD studies are useful for determining the effects a drug produces over the tested dose or concentration range. Species-specific differences in the PD of a drug can occur, therefore extrapolation between species may not be accurate. If not accounted for, PK differences can lead to inaccurate PD results, so both PK and PD data are needed to make accurate dose recommendations for clinical patients and clinical studies.

Clinical experience and case reports or series may not provide accurate data because of the difficulties in working with many zoologic companion animal species. Controlled clinical studies based on PK and PD studies and data are the best source of species-specific dose recommendations. Placebo-controlled, randomized, and blinded clinical studies provide the best data for dosing recommendations, but are rarely performed in veterinary species including zoologic companion animal species. Clinicians, research scientists, industry, and government agencies need to work together in order to provide the best data, and subsequently the best drug dosage recommendations, for nondomestic species because there are very few data currently available for the large number of animal species that require veterinary care, the rarity of some of these species, and the value (financial, emotional, and ecological) of maintaining the health and well-being of these species.

REFERENCES

1. Machin KL, Tellier LA, Lair S, et al. Pharmacodynamics of flunixin and ketoprofen in mallard ducks (*Anas platyrhynchos*). J Zoo Wildl Med 2001;32:222–9.
2. Metacam (meloxicam). Freedom of information summary. NADA 141–219.
3. Savides MC, Oehme FW, Nash SL, et al. The toxicity and biotransformation of single doses of acetaminophen in dogs and cats. Toxicol Appl Pharmacol 1984;74:26–34.
4. Toutain PL, Bousquet-Mélou A. Plasma terminal half-life. J Vet Pharmacol Ther 2004;27:427–39.
5. Uhrig SR, Papich MG, KuKanich B, et al. Pharmacokinetics and pharmacodynamics of morphine in llamas. Am J Vet Res 2007;68:25–34.
6. Seymour RA, Williams FM, Ward A, et al. Aspirin metabolism and efficacy in postoperative dental pain. Br J Clin Pharmacol 1984;17:697–701.
7. Benedek IH, Joshi AS, Pieniaszek HJ, et al. Variability in the pharmacokinetics and pharmacodynamics of low dose aspirin in healthy male volunteers. J Clin Pharmacol 1995;35:1181–6.
8. Sevoflo (sevoflurane). Freedom of information summary. NADA 141–103.
9. Riviere JE. Introduction. In Comparative pharmacokinetics: principles, techniques and applications. Ames (IA): Iowa State University Press; 1999. p. 3–10.
10. Souza MJ, Greenacre CB, Cox SK. Pharmacokinetics of orally administered tramadol in domestic rabbits (*Oryctolagus cuniculus*). Am J Vet Res 2008;69(8):979–82.
11. Yu S, Zhang X, Sun Y, et al. Pharmacokinetics of buprenorphine after intravenous administration in the mouse. J Am Assoc Lab Anim Sci 2006;45:12–6.
12. KuKanich B, Huff D, Riviere JE, et al. Naïve averaged, naïve pooled, and population pharmacokinetics of orally administered marbofloxacin in juvenile harbor seals. J Am Vet Med Assoc 2007;230:390–5.
13. Martín-Jiménez T, Riviere JE. Population pharmacokinetics in veterinary medicine: potential use for therapeutic drug monitoring and prediction of tissue residues. J Vet Pharmacol Ther 1998;21:167–89.

14. Riviere JE. Interspecies extrapolations. In: Comparative pharmacokinetics: principles, techniques and applications. Ames (IA): Iowa State University Press; 1999. p. 296–307.
15. Riviere JE, Martin-Jimenez T, Sundlof SF, et al. Interspecies allometric analysis of the comparative pharmacokinetics of 44 drugs across veterinary and laboratory animal species. J Vet Pharmacol Ther 1997;20:453–63.
16. Martinez M, Mahmood I, Hunter RP. Allometric scaling of clearance in dogs. J Vet Pharmacol Ther 2009;32:411–6.
17. KuKanich B, Papich M, Huff D, et al. Comparison of amikacin pharmacokinetics in a killer whale (*Orcinus orca*) and a beluga whale (*Delphinapterus leucas*). J Zoo Wildl Med 2004;35:179–84.
18. Maxwell LK, Jacobson ER. Allometric basis of enrofloxacin scaling in green iguanas. J Vet Pharmacol Ther 2008;31:9–17.
19. Mealey KL. Therapeutic implications of the MDR-1 gene. J Vet Pharmacol Ther 2004;27:257–64.
20. Mosher CM, Court MH. Comparative and veterinary pharmacogenomics. Handb Exp Pharmacol 2010;199:49–77.
21. Bulka A, Kouya PF, Böttiger Y, et al. Comparison of the antinociceptive effect of morphine, methadone, buprenorphine and codeine in two substrains of Sprague-Dawley rats. Eur J Pharmacol 2004;492:27–34.
22. Paronis CA, Holtzman SG. Increased analgesic potency of mu agonists after continuous naloxone infusion in rats. J Pharmacol Exp Ther 1991;259:582–9.
23. Le Bars D, Gozariu M, Cadden SW. Animal models of nociception. Pharmacol Rev 2001;53:597–652.
24. Bardo MT, Hughes RA. Shock-elicited flight response in chickens as an index of morphine analgesia. Pharmacol Biochem Behav 1978;9:147–9.
25. Paul-Murphy JR, Brunson DB, Miletic V. Analgesic effects of butorphanol and buprenorphine in conscious African grey parrots (*Psittacus erithacus erithacus* and *Psittacus erithacus timneh*). Am J Vet Res 1999;60:1218–21.
26. Sladky KK, Krugner-Higby L, Meek-Walker E, et al. Serum concentrations and analgesic effects of liposome-encapsulated and standard butorphanol tartrate in parrots. Am J Vet Res 2006;67:775–81.
27. Kanui TI, Hole K. Morphine and pethidine antinociception in the crocodile. J Vet Pharmacol Ther 1992;15:101–3.
28. Sladky KK, Miletic V, Paul-Murphy J, et al. Analgesic efficacy and respiratory effects of butorphanol and morphine in turtles. J Am Vet Med Assoc 2007;230:1356–62.
29. Peckham EM, Traynor JR. Comparison of the antinociceptive response to morphine and morphine-like compounds in male and female Sprague-Dawley rats. J Pharmacol Exp Ther 2006;316:1195–201.
30. Sladky KK, Kinney ME, Johnson SM. Analgesic efficacy of butorphanol and morphine in bearded dragons and corn snakes. J Am Vet Med Assoc 2008;233:267–73.
31. Williams DG, Dickenson A, Fitzgerald M, et al. Developmental regulation of codeine analgesia in the rat. Anesthesiology 2004;100:92–7.
32. Sato C, Sakai A, Ikeda Y, et al. The prolonged analgesic effect of epidural ropivacaine in a rat model of neuropathic pain. Anesth Analg 2008;106:313–20.
33. Cole GA, Paul-Murphy J, Krugner-Higby L, et al. Analgesic effects of intramuscular administration of meloxicam in Hispaniolan parrots (*Amazona ventralis*) with experimentally induced arthritis. Am J Vet Res 2009;70:1471–6.
34. Paul-Murphy JR, Krugner-Higby LA, Tourdot RL. Evaluation of liposome-encapsulated butorphanol tartrate for alleviation of experimentally induced arthritic pain in green-cheeked conures (*Pyrrhura molinae*). Am J Vet Res 2009;70:1211–9.

35. KuKanich B, Lascelles BD, Riviere JE, et al. Pharmacokinetic-pharmacody-namics modeling of morphine in dogs. J Vet Intern Med 2007;21:617.

36. Hug CC Jr, Murphy MR, Rigel EP, et al. Pharmacokinetics of morphine injected intravenously into the anesthetized dog. Anesthesiology 1981;54:38–47.

37. Shen DD, Artru AA, Adkison KK. Principles and applicability of CSF sampling for the assessment of CNS drug delivery and pharmacodynamics. Adv Drug Deliv Rev 2004;56:1825–57.

38. KuKanich B, Lascelles BD, Papich MG. Pharmacokinetics of morphine and plasma concentrations of morphine-6-glucuronide following morphine adminis-tration to dogs. J Vet Pharmacol Ther 2005;28:371–6.

39. Morphine sulfate [Package Insert]: Roxane Laboratories. NDA 022207.

40. KuKanich B, Lascelles BD, Papich MG. Use of a von Frey device for evaluation of pharmacokinetics and pharmacodynamics of morphine after intravenous admin-istration as an infusion or multiple doses in dogs. Am J Vet Res 2005;66:1968–74.

41. Lucas AN, Firth AM, Anderson GA, et al. Comparison of the effects of morphine administered by constant-rate intravenous infusion or intermittent intramuscular injection in dogs. J Am Vet Med Assoc 2001;218:884–91.

42. Sarton E, Romberg R, Dahan A. Gender differences in morphine pharmacoki-netics and dynamics. Adv Exp Med Biol 2003;523:71–80.

43. Kalvass JC, Olson ER, Cassidy MP, et al. Pharmacokinetics and pharmacody-namics of seven opioids in P-glycoprotein-competent mice: assessment of unbound brain EC50, u and correlation of in vitro, preclinical, and clinical data. J Pharmacol Exp Ther 2007;323:346–55.

44. Garcia-Villar R, Toutain PL, Alvinerie M, et al. The pharmacokinetics of xylazine hydrochloride: an interspecific study. J Vet Pharmacol Ther 1981;4:87–92.

45. Rompun (xylazine). Freedom of Information. NADA 047–956.

46. Gopal S, Tzeng TB, Cowan A. Characterization of the pharmacokinetics of bupre-norphine and norbuprenorphine in rats after intravenous bolus administration of buprenorphine. Eur J Pharm Sci 2002;15:287–93.

47. Abbo LA, Ko JC, Maxwell LK, et al. Pharmacokinetics of buprenorphine following intravenous and oral transmucosal administration in dogs. Vet Ther 2008;9:83–93.

48. Ingvast-Larsson C, Svartberg K, Hydbring-Sandberg E, et al. Clinical pharma-cology of buprenorphine in healthy, lactating goats. J Vet Pharmacol Ther 2007;30:249–56.

49. Kuhlman JJ Jr, Lalani S, Magluilo J Jr, et al. Human pharmacokinetics of intrave-nous, sublingual, and buccal buprenorphine. J Anal Toxicol 1996;20:369–78.

50. R Hanselmann, CI Mosley, CM Mosley, et al. Pharmacokinetics of buprenorphine in alpacas (Lama pacos) after intravenous and intramuscular administration. In: Proceedings of the 10th World Congress of Veterinary Anaesthesia. Glasgow (UK), August 31–September 4, 2009. p. 83.

51. Messenger KM, Davis JL, LaFevers BM, et al. The pharmacokinetics of intravenous and intramuscular buprenorphine in the horse. J Vet Intern Med 2009;23:785.

Fish Analgesia: Pain, Stress, Fear Aversion, or Nociception?

E. Scott Weber III, VMD, MSc (Distinction) Aquatic Pathobiology/Veterinary Science

KEYWORDS

• Fish • Stress • Analgesia • Neopallium • Nociception

Fish represent the largest class of vertebrate animals with more than 31,000 known species. The author estimates over 3000 species of these animals are used for a variety of purposes such as a protein source for humans and other animals, recreational and commercial fishing, companion animals, display animals, and research. To meet the ever increasing demands placed on fish, aquatic animal medicine is growing to help support veterinary needs for aquaculture, companion animal medicine, conservation medicine, laboratory animal medicine, zoo and aquarium medicine, ecosystem health, and wild fisheries for sport, recreation, restocking, and protection of endangered species. The increasing use of fish resources and a greater understanding of aquatic animal medicine demands providing evidence-based veterinary care for these animals. Because fish are aquatic as well as being pokilothermic, there are several unique anatomic and physiologic considerations that must be understood when working with these animals. Veterinarians need to adapt methodologies for examining, performing diagnostics, and treating fish patients to decrease stress, decrease fear, and avoid and/or decrease nociception. Recently several works have been published on the topic of fish anesthesia and analgesia in laboratory animal medicine, and these contributions are highly recommended for veterinarians seeking to get more information on these topics.[1,2] This article briefly defines stress, reviews and compares fish neuroanatomic pathways associated with nociception, discusses behavioral observations, summarizes current use of analgesics for fish patients, and concludes with the ongoing controversy regarding pain on this topic. With increasing concern on animal welfare in Europe and North America, veterinarians will also have a vital role contributing to objective research for better understanding the short- and long-term consequences of noxious stimuli as related to health and well-being for fish, reptiles, amphibians, and invertebrates.[3,4]

The author has nothing to disclose.
VM: Medicine and Epidemiology, University of California Davis School of Veterinary Medicine, 2108 Tupper Hall, Davis, CA 95616, USA
E-mail address: epweber@ucdavis.edu

STRESS IN FISH

Although there is more and more research being conducted using fish, stress is poorly defined for this and other classes of pokilothermic vertebrate and invertebrate animals. Homeostasis for fish patients refers to overall biologic and physiologic balance, or to the well-being of the host in its environmental conditions. Veterinarians try to maintain this balance and/or attempt to correct imbalances when presented with a fish patient. Barton and Iwama[5] defined stress as any event or action that challenged the homeostasis of the nearly resting animal. There are numerous studies, and it is well accepted that fish respond to stress with physiologic similarities and differences to other higher and lower vertebrates. Stress for fish patients involves a complicated integration of the animal and its environment. These stressors can serve to threaten or disturb the animal's homeostasis and cause a cascade of physiologic responses meant to be adaptive or compensatory.[6]

Overall disruption of normal physiology can lead to disease and is dependent on the individual's health, as well as intensity and duration of the stress or stressors. Fish disease can be most simply defined as an overall failure of the animal or animals to thrive. Some of the more common stressors identified for fish patients include: changes in either chemical or physical water quality conditions (water temperature, pH, alkalinity, salinity, DO); accumulation of nitrogenous waste in water; other environmental pollution; handling; transport; excess noise; poor/inadequate nutrition; overstocking; aggression; predation; infectious disease (parasitic, bacterial, viral, fungal); and many others. These stressors can invoke primary, secondary, and tertiary responses.[5] The fish neuroendocrine pathways for stress are very similar to other vertebrates, and they rely on the adrenergic system and the hypothalamic pituitary-interrenal (HPI) axis. The HPI axis is activated in response to stressors or noxious stimuli, and begins a central mediated cascade of events triggered by corticotropin-releasing factor (CRF) in all vertebrates studied to date.[7] When fish respond to stress acting on primary receptors or through a nerve-mediated motor response, a primary cascade begins to elicit an alarm response for fight or flight, with stimulation of the central nervous system (CNS) causing the hypothalamus and pituitary to release adrenocorticotropic hormone (ACTH).[8,9] Sympathetic neurons also send impulses to the teleost analogue for adrenal tissue that are called chromaffin cells. Chromaffin cells are grouped in clusters and scattered throughout the posterior kidney and posterior cardinal vein to release catecholamines such as epinephrine and norepinephrine. Simultaneously, the HPI axis causes release of corticosteroids from interrenal tissue also located within the posterior kidney, which are distributed throughout the bloodstream and cause physiologic changes, allowing the animal to respond.[8–11]

The consequence of the primary response can lead to secondary responses for resistance and adaptation if the stress duration persists, as many of the steroids can have longer-term effects than the initial catecholamine release. These secondary responses, as a result of circulating cortisol and catecholamines, can result in increased cardiac output, metabolic rate, respiration, plasma free fatty acids, lactic acidosis, and hematocrit, and have a varying effect on liver glycolysis and electrolyte balance.[12–16]

Tertiary responses are the result of chronic stress leading to physiologic exhaustion and can have long-term consequences, negatively affecting teleost immune function, locomotion/swimming, metabolism, reproduction, growth rate, behavior, and overall survival.[5,12,17–19]

By understanding the general stress response in fish, veterinarians will be able to assess many nonspecific signs of fish in distress marked by behavioral changes, anorexia, swimming, increased respiratory rate, increased heart rate, decreased body condition/condition factor, and changes in complete blood counts, hematocrit, glucose, and electrolyte values. Given the consequences of tertiary stress on fish patients, every effort should be made to manage and alleviate stressors in clinically ill patients when handling, diagnosing, treating, and maintaining fish patients for treatment, hospitalization, and quarantine. To ameliorate stress from the general examination through subsequent hospitalization for the numerous species that may be encountered, veterinarians should use practical husbandry solutions specific to the species, which may include decreasing water temperature, adding 1 to 3 ppt of sodium chloride to freshwater fishes, decreasing salinity for marine fish by 3–5 ppt, fasting before transport or procedures, reducing stocking densities, decreasing anesthetic time, and/or providing hide boxes or artificial plant material.[16,20] Not all anesthetic agents, sedatives, and analgesics used in fish medicine may have an effect on the stress cascade as described. Some agents may cause corticosteriod or catecholamine release when used, such as observed in Atlantic salmon (Salmo salar), Atlantic cod (Gadus morhua), and Atlantic halibut (Hippoglossus hippoglossus) with benzocaine, MS-222, metomidate, and isoeugenol.[21]

FISH NEUROANATOMY

Neuroanatomy is largely conserved among vertebrate animals within the peripheral nervous system and CNS.[22] A comprehensive discussion of fish neuroanatomy can be found in other publications.[23–25] A great deal more research needs to be completed, given the diversity of species in this class of vertebrates.

The peripheral nervous system consists of somatic and autonomic divisions, with the former responsible for motor skills and the latter being further subdivided into the sympathetic, parasympathetic, and enteric. The somatic nervous system controls voluntary body movements and maintains the body in its surroundings based on input from the various sensory systems. Divisions of the autonomic nervous system include the sympathetic nervous system, to which most often is attributed the "fight or flight" response that controls the response to stressful stimuli, and the parasympathetic nervous system that tries to be an antagonist to this response, conserving energy.

The peripheral nervous system is responsible for transmitting stimuli detected by nociceptors to the CNS. Nociceptors are bare axon nerve endings that are modified and specialized to detect temperature, pressure, and/or chemoreception terminating at the spinal nerves. Two types of polymodal fibers have been described in fish, namely A-delta fibers (Aδ fibers) and C fibers.[26] Aδ fibers are thin, myelinated, and can conduct information at moderate to fast speeds. These nerve fibers are afferent, detecting noxious stimuli and evoking immediate withdrawal from stimuli. By contrast, C fibers are unmyelinated and have slow conduction velocity, but respond to a stronger intensity of stimulus and are responsible for the dull, peracute and chronic, pain. Polymodal C fibers can adapt to a variety of physiologic changes with responses to hypoxia, hypercapnea, hyperthermia, hypothermia, hypoglycemia, hyperosmolarity, hypoosmolarity, and lactic acidosis.[27] Of the 3 major classes of fish, Osteichthyes (bony fishes) have both types of fibers although it is reported that Aδ fibers are a predominant type[28,29]; only Aδ fibers have been identified in Chrondrichthyes (elasmobranchs),[30] whereas the Agnatha (hagfishes and lamprey) primarily have C-type fibers.[31]

Nociceptive signals are transmitted from the nociceptors through the peripheral nerves, and are relayed via nerves of the spinothalamic and trigeminal tract in similar fashion to other vertebrates.[29,32] These nerves then relay information to the brain for processing.

The CNS of fish contains a spinal cord, medulla oblongata, and the brain, divided into telencephalon, diencephalon, mesencephalon, and cerebellum. Nociceptive processing occurs primarily in the forebrain that includes the diencephalon and telencephalon, with the former divided into epithalamus, thalamus, and hypothalamus, and the latter cerebral hemispheres. In fish, similar to other vertebrates, nociception travels from the peripheral nerves via the spinal nerves, and is relayed through the spinal cord to the thalamus. The thalamus is connected to the telencephalon via multiple connections through the gray matter pallium, which has been demonstrated to receive nerve relays for noxious and mechanical stimulu.[33] Some notable differences in the fish telencephalon are a thin roof plate and general lack of ventricle and ventricular sulcus.[23] Although there are differences in brain structure, it has been demonstrated that certain species of fish are able to process nociceptive responses in the brain, as demonstrated in comparisons between goldfish (Carassius auratus) and rainbow trout (Oncorhynchus mykiss) showing both species had neuronal activity in the spinal cord, cerebellum, tectum, and telencephalon from mechanoreceptive and nociceptive stimuli; and further demonstrating that all fish are not the same, goldfish having exhibited greater neuronal activity than rainbow trout when receiving noxious versus mechanical stimuli.[33]

In endothermic vertebrates the general pain pathway involves complex interactions of peripheral nerves, spinal cord, and brain. These interactions begin with nociceptor nerve endings modified and specialized to detect temperature, pressure, and/or chemoreception, which are bare-axoned and terminate in the spinal cord. A painful stimulus detected by the nociceptors travels via electrical impulse through the spinal cord where other specialized neurons serve to relay, ignore, or amplify the response to the brain. These impulses then travel to the thalamus, and are sent to the cerebral cortex and neocortex or limbic center. These 2 areas then elicit response consisting of a coordinated motor response from the cerebral cortex and an emotional response from the neocortex. This emotional response is what is largely accepted as allowing conscious thought and ultimately pain.[26,27] The 6-layer neocortex or neopallium is the outer layer of the cerebral hemispheres, and 1 of the 3 components of the cerebral cortex (neocortex, archicortex, and paleocortex). Reptiles were thought to have first evolved the neocortex in vertebrates, but the neopallium is absent in amphibians and fish.[34] In fish the archipallium is the largest part of the cerebrum, and is believed to have developed into the hippocampus in other vertebrates.[35] These differences in brain function between classes of vertebrates, in addition to greater variation among fish species, complicate functional and physiologic comparisons with inference to the human concept of pain. Because fish and amphibians lack a neopallium, this difference is the foundation for debate among researchers over whether these animals feel pain, and is discussed briefly in this article.

Neurotransmitters

The physical networks of nerves are the highway for these connections to travel from the periphery and be processed centrally, but they are heavily dependent on both local and systemic effects of several biochemical neurotransmitters or neuromodulators. These substances include endogenous opioid compounds, opiate-related compounds, substance P, and Mauthner cells, and are produced in various anatomic locations, and act on receptors in the brain and spinal cord. Substance P is a neuropeptide with receptors found throughout the CNS. Substance P and other sensory neuropeptides may be involved with neurogenic inflammation and are released from peripheral nerve fibers at the site of noxious stimuli in response to injury or infection.[36] In 1956, substance P was discovered in the intestine and the brain of fish and was shown to have depressive, hyperalgesic, and morphine antagonist effects on the CNS.[37,38] Evidence for endogenous opioids and opioid receptors began with discovery of β-endorphin–like immunoreactive substance in the brain of *Boops boops* and understanding that these compounds are involved with a hypophysial regulatory factor or neuromodulatory agent, similar to other vertebrates.[39] All 4 main opioid receptor types (delta, kappa, mu, and NOP) were found to be conserved in vertebrates, even in primitive jawless fishes (agnathastoma).[40] In addition, endogenous opioids were noted to affect serum gonadotropic hormone (GtH) levels in male goldfish, and were identified during reproduction for male brown bullhead catfish, *Ictalurus nebulosus* Lesueur.[41,42] The endogenous opioid peptide system in male brown bullhead catfish is characterized by naloxone binding and the response to naloxone during the annual reproductive cycle. More direct evidence for the presence of endogenous opioid peptides was revealed using immunohistochemistry to locate α-melanotrophin in the pars intermedia of the Australian lungfish *Neoceratodus forsteri*, and met-enkephalin in the CNS of teleosts *Anguilla rostrata* and *Oncorhynchus kisutch*.[43,44] The GABA$_A$ receptor ionically binds γ-aminobutyric acid (GABA) to inhibit neurotransmission in the CNS. The effects mediated by this ligand-gated ion channel make it a target for benzodiazepine (BZ) tranquilizers. These BZ binding sites have also been identified and partially characterized in whole brain membranes of male rainbow trout.[45] Mauthner cells are special cells in teleost fish, believed to initiate escape responses.[46] The presence or absence of Mauthner cells shows a clear correlation and dramatic differences in fast-start behavior when compared in several species of puffer fish.[47]

OBJECTIVE AND SUBJECTIVE BEHAVIORAL EVIDENCE OF PAIN IN FISH

Although some of the evidence for whether fish feel pain is found in neuroanatomy and neurophysiology, behavior is commonly used to discern pain in other animals and human infants. When monitoring fish patients for clinical signs of distress, some considerations include the subjective assessments of body orientation and swimming, feeding, hiding, and/or spatial positioning (near aeration or heater). Additional parameters are more medically specific and objective, for example, environmental quality parameters, heart rate, opercular or respiratory rate, lethargy, fin clamping, darkening, diagnostic values (eg, complete blood count and blood chemistries), and/or physical examination findings.

When examining a fish patient, vital signs are as critical as for mammalian patients. It has been well demonstrated that increased respiratory rate and cardiac output can be observed when brown trout (*Salmo trutta*) are subjected to either handling stress[48] or rainbow trout to noxious stimuli simulated by bee venom or acetic acid solution into the lip.[49]

Much of the controversy about identifying stress, pain, and/or distress in fish surrounds a lack of critical and comprehensive clinical data for a majority of species. Noticing changes in diagnostic results for fish is challenging, as normal baselines for many species are not readily available. When abnormalities are detected it is important to place this in the context of the entire physical examination, environmental quality parameters, and observation for a potentially ill fish patient. Several changes in blood chemistry have been observed in largemouth bass (*Micropterus salmoides*) from tournament-caught fish in a catch-and-release tournament that were sampled within 5 minutes after official tournament weigh-in.[50] Several chemistry parameters for these animals were significantly greater than controls, including plasma cortisol, glucose, sodium, and potassium, and large changes in metabolic status for these fish included major reductions in the muscle energy stores phosphocreatine, adenosine triphosphate, and glycogen, and large increases in muscle and plasma lactate concentrations.[50]

Fish can exhibit abnormal behavior when ill, and a variety of these behaviors have been documented. Rainbow trout treated with noxious stimuli injected into their lips can also have unusual behavior such as rocking on either pectoral fin from side to side, and also rubbing their lips into the gravel and against the sides of the tank.[49]

One of the most common subjective reasons for providing pain medication in fish patients is to eliminate anorexia. Inappetence or anorexia is a common finding of compromised fish patients, and can be a complication after anesthesia, after diagnostic procedures, and/or following surgery. There is greater evidence for the stress mechanisms in causing fish to become anorectic. In rainbow trout chronic plasma cortisol elevation affected individual appetite with subsequent decreases in growth rate, condition factor, and food conversion efficiency.[51] Using CNS injections of CRF and the related peptide, urotensin I (UI) in goldfish, appetite suppression occurred in a dose-related manner, and after intracoelomic CRF receptor antagonists were implanted in fish as glucocorticoid receptor antagonists, the blocked receptors reversed the appetite-suppressing effects previously observed.[52] Ammonia is toxic to fish, and many species exhibit anorexia when exposed to high ammonia levels. Investigators using rainbow trout to understand the appetite-suppressing effects of high environmental ammonia analyzed food intake after exposing fish to various doses of NH3, and have noted that appetite decreased in a dose-dependent manner after 24 h of ammonia exposure.[53] In these animals brain serotonin (5-HT) was the key neuromodulator associated with this change of anorectic behavior due to high ammonia.[53]

There are also numerous researchers dedicating time to understanding avoidance behavior exhibited by fish, which is relevant to the current debate and discussion. An example of behavioral responses to acute noxious stimuli comparing rainbow trout with goldfish involved observing animals after administering electric shocks of 2 different intensities directly to the skin; goldfish demonstrated spatially cued shock avoidance with significantly improved shock-avoidance learning, whereas trout displayed a difference when a conspecific was presented and remained in the area of the conspecific when it was being subjected to the stimuli.[54]

ANALGESIA IN FISH

In brief, anesthesia and/or sedation can be administered via bath, orally, or via injection using a variety of substances that have been used to anesthetize fish including ethanol, diethylether, benzodiazepines, halothane, lidocaine, benzocaine, tricaine methanesulfonate, eugenol, ketamine, medetomidine, propofol, carbon dioxide, iso-eugenol, oxygen, and many other substances.[55] In the United States there is one federally approved anesthetic agent, tricaine methanesulfonate, also called MS222, which is added to water as a bath application. Tricaine methanesulfonate is used for a variety of species, and many teleost and elasmobranch fish can be induced at a dose of 75 to 110 mg/L.[55] The reader is referred to a recent review by Ross and Ross[56] on anesthetic and sedative techniques for aquatic animals. It should be noted, as previously stated in this article, that anesthetic agents in fish may not always provide analgesic effects and can increase or have no effect on the stress response of fish.

Nociception is the response of an animal to a noxious stimulus, and is a current topic in research circles and for animal welfare concerns related to fish.[57–63] Research pharmacology that provides analgesic drugs and dosages for fish patients is scarce in veterinary literature; however, most veterinarians assume that fish behave negatively to noxious stimulus, and use analgesics to ameliorate the nociceptive response or pain perceived in these animals. Comparisons have been made using intraoperative administration of the opiate butorphanol (0.4 mg/kg) or the nonsteroidal anti-inflammatory analgesic ketoprofen (2 mg/kg) in koi (Cyprinus carpio).[64] In this study the untreated controls and ketoprofen-treated fish had decreased activity and appetite after surgery, in contrast to the butorphanol-treated group; in addition, decreased creatinine kinase was noted in the ketoprofen group, suggesting a mild behavioral sparing effect of butorphanol and reduced muscle damage from the ketoprofen.[64] Using morphine, winter flounder (Pseudopleuronectes americanus) given a noxious stimulus such as the injection of acetic acid resulted without an acute change in cardiac response, but subsequent long-term increases of heart rate and cardiac output were noted.[65] When morphine was administered to rainbow trout that were injected with a noxious substance in the lip, these animals exhibited less abnormal behavior and had a decreased respiratory rate compared with untreated controls.[66] Similarly, when rainbow trout were given an opiate antagonist after morphine, administration of electrical impulses to produce agitated swimming responses resulted in significantly reduced analgesic effects compared with controls, in a dose-dependent fashion from 20 to 150 minutes.[67]

In common carp (Cyprinus carpio) a prolonged analgesic response was observed when tramadol, an agonist of the opioid mu receptor, was given before applying a noxious electrical stimulus. The effect was observed to be both dose dependent and to last for 2 hours, with fish maintaining normal swimming and their normal behavioral repertoire compared with controls that did not receive tramadol.[68] Unlike teleosts, elasmobranchs such as chain dogfish (Scyliorhinus retifer), when administered multiple doses of each of the analgesics (0.25, 0.5, 1.0, 2.5, and 5.0 mg/kg butorphanol and 1.0, 1.5, 2.0, and 4.0 mg/kg ketoprofen) before undergoing anesthesia did not have a significant reduction of anesthetic concentration with MS-222.[69]

Many nonsteroidal anti-inflammatory drugs (NSAIDs) and opiates are available to veterinarians, such as carprofen, meloxicam, ketoprofen, flunixin meglumine, butorphanol, tramadol, morphine, and buprenorphine.[55] Because pharmacokinetic studies are not available for many of these compounds for the variety of fish species commonly seen as patients, empirical dosing may be used. The most common application for analgesia in fish is for surgery, trauma, cutaneous ulceration, or inflammatory lesions.[70] Some drug doses commonly used are shown in **Table 1**. No analgesics are currently approved in the United States for use in fish and these dosages are limited to several ornamental companion animal species, so they should be used cautiously and never in fish intended for human consumption.

PAIN IN FISH

The question of whether fish feel pain is extremely and pointedly relevant as veterinary expertise continues to offer a greater range of nonlethal diagnostic and treatment options for fish patients. It is a question posed by clients as well as the general public for a variety of reasons stemming from fish surgery to catch-and-release sport fishing, and from fish research to the evolving views on animal welfare. Whether fish feel pain is also increasingly debated among researchers, with the most publicized exchange on this issue being documented in the scientific literature between Drs Sneddon[49,58,66] and Rose.[59,63] These debates largely stem from the evolution and anatomy of the fish brain, which lacks a neopallium, the site where pain is thought to be perceived in higher homoeothermic vertebrates, as compared with other research on nociception, behavior, and opioid receptors and endogenous opioids conserved in fish.[71]

Table 1
Fish analgesic agents and dosages: commonly used analgesics in veterinary medicine that have been used in fish patients

Drug	Dose (mg/kg)	Route	Interval (hours)	References	Comments
Opioids					
Buprenorphine	Not recorded: 0.01–0.02 in cats and dogs			55	Wide range of safety and efficacy
Butorphanol	0.1–0.4	IM	24	55,64	Dose varies species to species with efficacy
Morphine	0.3	IM		70	Used in research; dose varies species to species
Oxymorphone	Not recorded				10× potency of morphine
Tramadol	5.0–10.0	PO	48–72	68	
NSAIDs and others					
Carprofen	2.0–4.0	IM	72–96	70	NSAID side effects; gastric ulceration observed in sand tiger shark (*Carcharias taurus*) with long-term use
Flunixin	0.25–0.5	IM	72–96	55	
Ketoprofen	2.0	IM		64,69	
Meloxicam	0.1–0.2	IM	24–48	70	

Abbreviations: IM, intramuscular; NSAID, nonsteroidal anti-inflammatory drug; PO, by mouth.

Whether fish feel pain, are simply fear aversive, or are experiencing nociception to any noxious stimulus caused from disease, poor husbandry, handling, or transport, it is a veterinary responsibility to help ameliorate this stress and/or distress in a similar way to practical veterinary solutions employed for other livestock, pet, laboratory animal, and wild populations.

ACKNOWLEDGMENTS

I want to dedicate this article to all my fish patients over the years that have allowed me to evolve and grow in my knowledge of aquatic animal medicine, and also to Dr Greg Lewbart, who has mentored me over the years and first inspired me to pursue my veterinary goals in aquatic animal health.

REFERENCES

1. Stoskopf M, Posner LP. Anesthesia and restraint of laboratory fish. In: Fish RE, Danneman PJ, Brown M, editors. Anesthesia and analgesia in laboratory animals. 2nd edition. London: Academic Press; 2008. p. 519–34.
2. Smith SA. Pain and distress in fish issue. ILAR J 2009;50(4):327–415.

3. FAWC. Report on the welfare of farmed fish. Surrey: Farm Animal Welfare Council. 1996. Available at: http://www.fawc.org.uk/reports/fish/fishrtoc.htm. Accessed August 6, 2010.

4. Yue S. An HSUS report: fish and pain perception. 2009. Available at: www.humanesociety.org/assets/pdfs/farm/hsus-fish-and-pain-perception.pdf. yue fish HSUS. Accessed August 6, 2010.

5. Barton BA, Iwama GK. Physiological changes in fish from stress in aquaculture with emphasis on the response and effects of corticosteroids. Annu Rev Fish Dis 1991;1:3–26.

6. Wendelaar Bonga SE. The stress response in fish. Physiol Rev 1997;77:591–625.

7. Denver RJ. Structural and functional evolution of vertebrate neuroendocrine stress systems. Trends in comparative endocrinology and neurobiology. Ann N Y Acad Sci 2009;1163:1–16.

8. Donaldson EM. The pituitary-interrenal axis as an indicator of stress in fish. In: Pickering AD, editor. Stress and fish. London: Academic; 1981. p. 11–47.

9. Reid SG, Bernier NJ, Perry SF. The adrenergic stress response in fish: control of catecholamine storage and release. Comp Biochem Physiol C Pharmacol Toxicol Endocrinol 1998;120:1–27.

10. Barton BA. Stress in fishes: a diversity of responses with particular reference to changes in circulating corticosteroids. Integr Comp Biol 2002;42:517–25.

11. Mommsen TP, Vijayan MM, Moon TW. Cortisol in teleosts: dynamics, mechanisms of action, and metabolic regulation. Rev Fish Biol Fish 1999;9:211–68.

12. Mazeaud MM, Mazeaud F. Adrenergic responses to stress in fish. In: Pickering AD, editor. Stress and fish. New York: Academic Press; 1981. p. 49–75.

13. Woodward CC, Strange RJ. Physiological stress responses in wild and hatchery-reared rainbow trout. Trans Am Fish Soc 1987;116:574–9.

14. Wedemeyer GA, Barton BA, McLeay DJ. Stress and acclimation. In: Schreck CB, Moyle PB, editors. Methods for fish biology. Bethesda (MD): American Fisheries Society; 1990. p. 451–89.

15. Ackerman PA, Forsyth RB, Mazur CF, et al. Stress hormones and the cellular stress response in salmonids. Fish Physiol Biochem 2000;23:327–36.

16. Wedemeyer GA, McLeay DJ. Methods for determining the tolerance of fishes to environmental stressors. In: Pickering AD, editor. Stress and fish. London: Academic Press; 1981. p. 247–75.

17. Iwama GK, Pickering AD, Sumpter JP, et al. Fish stress and health in aquaculture. Cambridge (UK): Cambridge University Press; 1997.

18. Maule AG, Tripp RA, Kaattari SL, et al. Stress alters immune function and disease resistance in chinook salmon (*Oncorhynchus tshawytscha*). J Endocrinol 1989; 120:135–42.

19. Barton BA, Morgan JD, Vijayan MM. Physiological and condition-related indicators of environmental stress in fish. In: Adams SM, editor. Biological indicators of aquatic ecosystem stress. Bethesda (MD): American Fisheries Society; 2002. p. 111–48.

20. Pickering AD, Pottinger TG. Stress response and disease resistance in salmonid fish: effects of chronic elevation of plasma cortisol. Fish Physiol Biochem 1989;7: 253–8.

21. Zahl IH, Kiessling A, Samuelsen OB, et al. Anesthesia induces stress in Atlantic salmon (*Salmo salar*), Atlantic cod (*Gadus morhua*) and Atlantic halibut (*Hippoglossus hippoglossus*). Fish Physiol Biochem 2009;36(3):719–30.

22. Butler AB, Hodos W, editors. Comparative vertebrate neuroanatomy: evolution and adaptation. 2nd edition. Hoboken (NJ): John Wiley & Sons, Inc; 2005. p. 73–89.

23. Bernstein JJ. Anatomy and physiology of the central nervous system. In: Hoar WS, Randall DJ, editors, Fish physiology, vol. iv. Orlando (FL): Academic Press; 1970. p. 2–90.
24. Butler AB. Nervous system. In: Ostrander GK, editor. The laboratory fish. London (UK): Elsevier Ltd; 2000. p. 129–49.
25. Bernier N, Van Der Kraak G, Farrell A, et al, editors, Fish physiology, fish neuro-endocrinology, vol. 28. Orlando (FL): Academic Press; 2009. p. 1–527.
26. Besson JM. The neurobiology of pain. Lancet 1999;353:1610–5.
27. Craig AD. Interoception: the sense of the physiological condition of the body. Curr Opin Neurobiol 2003;13(4):500–5.
28. Ashley PJ, Sneddon LU, McCrohan CR. Nociception in fish: stimulus-response properties of receptors on the head of trout *Oncorhynchus mykiss*. Brain Res 2007;1166:47–54.
29. Sneddon LU. Anatomical and electrophysiological analysis of the trigeminal nerve in a teleost fish, *Oncorhynchus mykiss*. Neurosci Lett 2002;319:167–71.
30. Coggeshall RE, Leonard RB, Applebaum ML, et al. Organisation of peripheral nerves of the Atlantic stingray, *Dasyatis sabina*. J Neurophysiol 1978;41:97–107.
31. Matthews G, Wickelgren WO. Trigeminal sensory neurons of the sea lamprey. J Comp Physiol A Neuroethol Sens Neural Behav Physiol 1978;123:329–33.
32. Murakami T, Ito H. Long ascending projections of the spinal dorsal horn in a teleost, *Sebastiscus marmoratus*. Brain Res 1985;346:168–70.
33. Dunlop R, Laming P. Mechanoreceptive and nociceptive responses in the central nervous system of goldfish (*Carassius auratus*) and trout (*Oncorhynchus mykiss*). J Pain 2005;6(9):561–8.
34. Dart RA. The dual structure of the neopallium: its history and significance. J Anat 1934;69(Pt 1):3–19.
35. Northcutt RG. Evolution of the telencephalon in nonmammals. Annu Rev Neurosci 1981;4:301–50.
36. Zubrzycka M, Janecka A, Substance P. Transmitter of nociception (minireview). Endocr Regul 2000;34(4):195–201.
37. Ostlund E, Von Euler US. Occurrence of a substance P-like polypeptide in fish intestine and brain. Br J Pharmacol Chemother 1956;11(3):323–5.
38. Zetler G. [Substance P, a polypeptide from the intestine and the brain, with depressive, hyperalgesic and morphine antagonist effects on CNS]. Naunyn Schmiedebergs Arch Exp Pathol Pharmakol 1956;228(6):513–38 [in German].
39. Vallarino M. Occurrence of β-endorphin-like immunoreactivity in the brain of the teleost, *Boops boops*. Gen Comp Endocrinol 1985;60(1):63–9.
40. Dreborg S, Rel Sundstrom G, Larsson TA, et al. Evolution of vertebrate opioid receptors. Proc Natl Acad Sci U S A 2008;105(40):15487–92.
41. Rosenblum PM, Callard IP. Endogenous opioid peptide system in male brown bullhead catfish, *Ictalurus nebulosus* Lesueur: characterization of naloxone binding and the response to naloxone during the annual reproductive cycle. J Exp Zool 1988;245(3):244–55.
42. Rosenblum PM, Peter RE. Evidence for the involvement of endogenous opioids in the regulation of gonadotropin secretion in male goldfish, *Carassius auratus*. Gen Comp Endocrinol 1989;73(1):21–7.
43. Dores RM, Joss JM. Immunological evidence for multiple forms of alpha-melano-trophin in the pars intermedia of the Australian lungfish *Neoceratodus forsteri*. Gen Comp Endocrinol 1988;71:468–74.
44. McDonald LK, Dores RM. Detection of met-enkephalin in the CNS of teleosts *Anguilla rostrata* and *Oncorhynchus kisutch*. Peptides 1991;12:541–7.

45. Wilkinson M, Wilkinson DA, Khan I, et al. Benzodiazepine receptors in fish brain: [3H]-flunitrazepam binding and modulatory effects of GABA in rainbow trout. Brain Res Bull 1983;10(3):301–3.

46. Eaton RC, Lee RK, Foreman MB. The Mauthner cell and other identified neurons of the brainstem escape network of fish. Prog Neurobiol 2001;63(4):467–85.

47. Greenwood K, Peichel CL, Zottoli SJ. Distinct startle responses are associated with neuroanatomical differences in pufferfishes. J Exp Biol 2010;213:613–20.

48. Laitinen M, Valtonen T. Cardiovascular, ventilatory and total activity responses of brown trout to handling stress. J Fish Biol 1994;45:933–42.

49. Sneddon LU, Braithwaite VA, Gentle MJ. Do fish have nociceptors? Evidence for the evolution of a vertebrate sensory system. Proc Biol Sci 2003;270(1520): 1115–21.

50. Suski CD, Killen SS, Morrissey MB, et al. Physiological changes in largemouth bass caused by live-release angling tournaments in southeastern Ontario. N Am J Fish Manag 2003;23:760–9.

51. Gregory TR, Wood CM. The effects of chronic plasma cortisol elevation on the feeding behaviour, growth, competitive ability, and swimming performance of juvenile rainbow trout. Physiol Biochem Zool 1999;72(3):286–95.

52. Bernier NJ, Peter RE. Appetite-suppressing effects of urotensin I and cortico-tropin-releasing hormone in goldfish (*Carassius auratus*). Neuroendocrinology 2001;73:248–60.

53. Ortega VA, Renner KJ, Bernier NJ. Appetite-suppressing effects of ammonia exposure in rainbow trout associated with regional and temporal activation of brain monoaminergic and CRF systems. J Exp Biol 2005;208:1855–66.

54. Dunlop R, Millsopp S, Laming P. Avoidance learning in goldfish (*Carassius auratus*) and trout (*Oncorhynchus mykiss*) and implications for pain perception. Appl Anim Behav Sci 2006;97(2):255–71.

55. Weber ES 3rd, Weisse C, Schwarz T, et al. Anesthesia, diagnostic imaging, and surgery of fish. Compend Contin Educ Vet 2009;31(2):E1–9 Online.

56. Ross L, Ross B. Anaesthetic and sedative techniques for aquatic animals. 3rd edition. Oxford (UK): Wiley-Blackwell; 2008.

57. Volpato GL. Challenges in assessing fish welfare. ILAR J 2009;50:329–37.

58. Sneddon LU. Pain perception in fish: indicators and endpoints. ILAR J 2009;50: 338–42.

59. Rose JD. The neurobehavioral nature of fishes and the question of awareness of pain. Rev Fish Sci 2002;10(1):1–38.

60. Ackerman PA, Morgan JD, Iwama GK. Anesthetics. CCAC guidelines on: the care and use of fish in research, teaching and testing. Available at: http://www.ccac.ca/en/CCAC_Programs/Guidelines_Policies/GDLINES/Fish/Fish%20Anesthetics%20-%20ENG.pdf. Ottawa (Canada): Canadian Council on Animal Care; 2005. Accessed August 6, 2010.

61. Chandroo KP, Yue S, Moccia RD. An evaluation of current perspectives on consciousness and pain in fishes. Fish Fish 2004;5:281–95.

62. Grandin T, Deesing M. Distress in animals: is it fear, pain, or physical stress? Manhattan Beach (CA): American Board of Veterinary Practitioners-Symposium; 2002. Available at: www.grandin.com/welfare/fear.pain.stress.html. Accessed August 6, 2010.

63. Rose J. A critique of the paper: "do fish have nociceptors: evidence for the evolution of a vertebrate sensory system" published in proceedings of the royal society: Biolog Sci 2003; 270(1520):1115–1121 by Sneddon, Braithwaite and Gentle. Available at: http://www.nal.usda.gov/awic/pubs/Fishwelfare/RoseC.pdf. Accessed 6 August 2010.

64. Harms CA, Lewbart GA, Swanson CR, et al. Behavioral and clinical pathology changes in koi carp (*cyprinus carpio*) subjected to anesthesia and surgery with and without intra-operative analgesics. Comp Med 2005;55(3):221–6.
65. Newby NC, Gamper AK, Stevens ED. Cardiorespiratory effects and efficacy of morphine sulfate in winter flounder (*Pseudopleuronectes americanus*). Am J Vet Res 2007;68(6):592–7.
66. Sneddon LU. The evidence for pain in fish: the use of morphine as an analgesic. Appl Anim Behav Sci 2003;83:153–62.
67. Ehrensing RH, Michell GF, Kastin AJ. Similar antagonism of morphine analgesia by mif-1 and naloxone in *Carassius auratus*. Pharmacol Biochem Behav 1982; 17:757–61.
68. Chervova LS, Lapshin DN. Opioid modulation of pain threshold in fish. Dokl Biol Sci 2000;375:590–1.
69. Davis MR, Mylniczenko N, Storms T, et al. Evaluation of intramuscular ketoprofen and butorphanol as analgesics in chain dogfish (*Scyliorhinus retifer*). Zoo Biol 2006;25:491–500.
70. Roberts HE. Anesthesia, analgesia, and euthanasia. In: Roberts HE, editor. Fundamentals of ornamental fish health. Ames (IA): Blackwell Publishing; 2010. p. 169.
71. Laming D. Brain mechanisms of behaviour in lower vertebrates. Cambridge (UK): Cambridge University Press; 1981. p. 7–79.

Analgesia in Amphibians: Preclinical Studies and Clinical Applications

Craig W. Stevens, PhD

KEYWORDS

• Analgesia • Amphibians • Opioid • Acetic acid test
• *Rana pipiens*

Analgesia is the selective loss of pain sensation leaving other cognitive, sensory, and motor functions intact and ideally, unaltered. General anesthesia is the loss of all sensory and motor function, and a total lack of consciousness and awareness. Both analgesia and anesthesia are defined by description of these states in humans; it is at best an educated guess whether these definitions can also be applied accurately to non-human animals or amphibians. Comparative neurology suggests that the potential for pain is less substantial in amphibians and other earlier-evolved vertebrates than in humans.[1–4]

There are very limited studies on either analgesia or anesthesia in amphibian species, and only a few agents are recommended for clinical use. Anesthesia studies can be done to determine appropriate pharmacologic agents and dosages by assessing simple measures like ability of an animal to right itself or to withdraw its limb from a strong forceps pinch,[5–9] but such studies will not be considered further here. By contrast, studies of analgesia are more difficult in amphibians as a validated assay is needed in which the animal exhibits a specific behavior in response to a potentially painful stimulus and in which that response is reduced by a potential analgesic agent. A well-validated alternative pain and analgesia model using *Rana pipiens* has been in use for more than 25 years[10,11]; however, in general, studies of analgesia in any non-mammalian species are surprisingly limited.[12,13] As discussed elsewhere, there are several reasons for the limited research on pain and analgesics using nonmammalian

This work was supported in part by Grant No. DA012248 from the National Institutes of Health. The author has nothing to disclose.
Department of Pharmacology & Physiology, Oklahoma State University-Center for Health Sciences, 1111 West 17th Street, Tulsa, OK 74107, USA
E-mail address: cw.stevens@okstate.edu

pain models, including the biased view of alternative models by funding agencies, dismissive regulations of nonmammalian species, and lack of a scientific and zoologic perspective by some scientists, veterinarians, and animal welfare experts.[14] This article reviews the nociceptive pathways and related systems in amphibians, summarizes the results of preclinical studies of analgesics in amphibian pain models, and provides clinical guidelines and rationale for the use of analgesics in amphibians.

NOCICEPTION AND PAIN IN AMPHIBIANS

Nociception is used to describe the transmission of noxious stimuli and subsequent processing up to the point in the brain whereby the pain experience, if present, is mediated. However, for ease of use and to make research findings accessible to a general audience, the term pain is generally used instead of nociception, and analgesia is used instead of antinociception in nonhuman animal studies. As our attitudes about animals are reflected by the language we use describing them and their possible attributes, word usage in this case is not a trivial point.[15] Most pain researchers accept this less precise usage of the words pain and analgesia (nociception and antinociception being too cumbersome and pedantic), but this does not necessarily imply that these researchers believe that the animals they treat or use for research experience pain as we do. It also does not mean that researchers using nonhuman animals believe that animals do not feel pain. In this regard, we must remain agnostic, using the best available science to guide our judgment. To think we know what an animal experiences or is feeling is not science but science fiction. The terms pain and analgesia are used here for convenience and in doing so make no assumptions as to the capacity of nonmammalian animals to experience pain.

The nociceptive pathways of amphibians were recently reviewed in detail.[16] In brief, there are no major differences between amphibian nociceptive afferents and those primary afferents of other vertebrates including mammals. Early electrophysiological work suggested that the detection of all noxious sensory stimuli, including chemical, was mediated exclusively by the same free nerve endings associated with thermal sensitivity in amphibians.[17] Amphibians, like mammals, possess both myelinated and unmyelinated afferent fibers running concurrently in mixed-fiber peripheral sensory nerves. These afferent fibers have been delineated into 3 general classes based on morphology, conduction velocities, latency of response, and action potential characteristics: large, heavily myelinated A fibers; small, thinly myelinated B fibers; and small, unmyelinated C fibers. Their characteristics correlate well with those observed in corresponding classes of somatic sensory afferents in mammals: $A\beta$, $A\delta$, and C fibers, respectively.[16] In studies that separated fibers both by conduction velocity and fiber diameter in amphibians, small slowly-conducting fibers transmitted the majority of all impulses induced by noxious heat, pinching, pin pricks, and the application of dilute acetic acid to the skin.[17,18] A recent study closely examined the nociceptive primary afferent fibers excited in the acetic acid test (see later discussion) and found that concentrations producing the behavioral response to the cutaneously applied acid solution evoked both $A\beta$ and C fibers to an equal extent.[19]

There is some uncertainty concerning the central terminations of primary afferent fibers within the amphibian spinal gray matter[20]; most, but not all studies indicate that sensory afferents from the skin terminate in areas of the dorsal field of the frog spinal cord that corresponds to mammalian laminae I to IV. It appears that in more recently evolved vertebrates, primary afferent fibers retract their ventral horn connections and become more restricted to the superficial laminae of the spinal dorsal horn.[21] This situation may reflect an overall vertebrate evolutionary vector to put more neurons in between reflex arcs to allow for finer control of responses and greater response modulation.

The primary afferent nerve fibers in mammals terminate in the dorsal horn of the spinal cord and release pain-signaling neurotransmitters such as substance P, calcitonin gene-related peptide, and glutamate. Using immunohistochemical techniques, these algogenic substances are readily identified in abundance in the spinal dorsal horn of amphibians.[22,23] In mammals, substance P and glutamate excite second-order neurons that have their cell bodies in the dorsal horn and send long fibers upward to form the ascending pain pathway.[24] Such second-order neurons within the dorsal horn that receive direct primary afferent input have not been identified in amphibians.[25] Also present in the mammalian spinal cord are endorphinergic neurons that release met-enkephalin, an endogenous opioid peptide, to act presynaptically to inhibit the release of substance P and postsynaptically to decrease the firing of the second-order pain neurons. Likewise, met-enkephalin, as well as opioid receptors, are abundant in the amphibian spinal cord.[10,16] In addition, using in situ hybridization to identify neurons expressing mRNA for met-enkephalin, endorphinergic neurons were identified throughout the brain and spinal cord of Rana pipiens.[26] Thus although the most detailed studies have only been performed in mammals, the existence of these key pain neurotransmitters and endogenous opioid peptides suggests that basic mechanisms of pain transmission and endogenous opioid peptides within the spinal cord are common in both amphibians and mammals. An important caveat to remember, however, is that the presence of opioid receptors and endorphins (met-enkephalin or β-endorphin) in the central nervous system of any vertebrate is not by itself supporting evidence that these animals feel pain, as some investigators suggest.[27–29] Endorphins and opioid binding sites are located in several organisms that do not have the capacity for anything like human pain and have very limited nervous systems, such as the cockroach, crab, and snail.[30–33]

Ascending nociceptive pathways in amphibians are unclear, as the location of second-order neurons in the spinal cord and the route of their fibers that carry this information to the brain are unknown.[34] Functional studies of evoked responses in supraspinal sites after specific noxious stimulation of peripheral fibers are lacking. A single study found that electrical stimulation of the sciatic nerve produces evoked potentials in posterior thalamic nuclei and primordial hippocampal structures in frogs.[35] However, the general sensory tracts from spinal neurons make direct connections with neuron groups farther toward the front of the brain as the phylogeny of vertebrates is ascended.[36] Throughout phylogeny, all the target sites of spinal tracts in the brain increase in complexity, specialization, and number of neurons, suggesting that even nociceptive messages to the thalamus in an amphibian and mammal may not be similar.

Cortical tissue, whether in limbic or cerebral regions, is a highly complex and laminated structure that is a relatively recent development in the evolution of the vertebrate nervous system. We know from human experience that decreasing the activity of cortical neurons by anesthesia or surgical lesion results in a loss of the full appreciation of pain; the patient reports an awareness of pain "but it no longer bothers them."[37] Recent studies using positron imaging techniques also show specific areas of the cortex activated by noxious stimuli in awake humans.[38] For these reasons, there is agreement among various scientific organizations that an intact cortex assists in the appreciation of pain.[39–41] It is likely that amphibians, without either a cerebral or limbic cortex, have a diminished potential for the appreciation of pain. Even the most rudimentary cerebral and limbic cortex does not appear until class Reptilia. In this sense, the use of amphibians may represent a "purer" model system for the study of nociception, possibly without the additional factors of learning and conditioning that can interfere with the accurate measurement of analgesia in mammals.[42]

PRECLINICAL STUDIES OF AMPHIBIAN ANALGESIA
Pain Models in Amphibians

The first successful algesiometric model developed in the amphibian was described by Pezalla,[43] who used dilute concentrations of cutaneously applied acetic acid and watched for a wiping response. Called the acetic acid test (AAT), a determination of the nociceptive threshold (NT), as signaled by the wiping response, was done by placing, with a Pasteur pipette, a single drop of acid on the dorsal surface of the frog's thigh. Testing began with the lowest concentration and proceeded with increasing concentrations until the NT was reached. The NT was defined as the lowest concentration of acid that caused the frog to vigorously wipe the treated leg with either hindlimb. To prevent tissue damage, the acetic acid was immediately wiped off with a gentle stream of distilled water once the animal responded or after 5 seconds if the animal failed to respond. If the animal failed to respond, testing continued with the next highest concentration of acetic acid on the opposite hindlimb. The wiping response in frogs, like the tail-flick in rodents, remains intact after a high spinal transection, demonstrating sufficient circuitry in the spinal cord to mediate this behavior.[44] The acetic acid stimulus excites primary afferent fibers consistent with nociceptive stimulation.[19,45] This wiping response has not been observed in the laboratory in the absence of noxious stimuli, and appears specific for assessing nociception. The wiping response is also the basis for much research on the motor systems of the amphibian spinal cord.[46]

Opioid Analgesia in Amphibians

Using the AAT, initial and ongoing studies of the analgesic effects of opioid administration in amphibians was conducted using nonselective opioid agonists, endogenous opioid peptides, and antagonists.[47–52] These studies showed that both exogenous opioid agonists and endogenous opioid peptides could raise the NT in amphibians by an action at an opioid receptor. Tolerance to the analgesic effects of daily morphine administration was documented[53] and stress-induced release of endogenous opioids was shown to produce analgesia in amphibians, which was potentiated by enkephalinase inhibitors.[54] Other behavioral studies include an investigation of the effects of opioids on noxious and nonnoxious sensory modalities,[55,56] an examination of agents acting on α_2-adrenergic receptors after systemic and spinal administration,[57,58] and studies aimed at determining the selectivity of opioid receptors in amphibians.[59–63]

Later results of systematic studies examining the analgesia of selective mu, delta, or kappa opioid agonists administered by different routes yielded an important finding: The relative analgesic potency of mu, delta, or kappa opioid agonists after systemic, intraspinal, or intracerebroventricular administration in amphibians was highly correlated with that observed in typical mammalian models and with the relative analgesic potency of opioid analgesics in human clinical studies.[64–67] These data established the amphibian model, using the AAT as a robust and predictive adjunct or alternative nonmammalian model for the testing of opioid analgesics.

Two other studies also used the AAT to examine the potential analgesic effects of opioids in ranid frogs. Using *Rana pipiens*, Terril-Robb and colleagues[27] demonstrated a dose-dependent analgesic effect of butorphanol, a mixed mu-kappa opioid receptor agent. Butorphanol has the logistical advantage that unlike the more potent opioids such as morphine, it is not a Schedule II agent and is therefore easier to obtain for veterinary use and to keep in animal facilities. Using the common European water frog, *Rana esculenta*, Benyhe and colleagues[68] confirmed the potency of morphine on the AAT and also showed that oxymorphazone, an analogue of oxymorphone that binds irreversibly to mu opioid receptors, produced a long-lasting analgesia up to 48 hours. **Table 1** provides a summary of the dosage range and effective dose (ED$_{50}$) values for the analgesic effect of opioid agonists used in behavioral studies of in *Rana pipiens* following systemic administration.

A recent study examined the potential analgesic effects of buprenorphine and butorphanol in another amphibian species, the Eastern red-spotted newt (*Notophthalmus viridescens*).[69] In this study, the AAT was not used but rather animals underwent bilateral forelimb amputation, and "analgesia" was assayed by changes in food consumption, spontaneous movement, and other nonspecific measures. There was a significant shortening of the time to resume normal behaviors following postoperative systemic administration of buprenorphine or bath application of butorphanol compared with animals receiving no postoperative agents. Finally, using the Japanese fire-belly newt (*Cynops pyrrhogaster*), administration of the neuropeptide RFamide produced an increase in the latency to withdrawal the newt's tail from a hot lamp (like the common tail-flick test used in rodents), which was blocked by the opioid antagonist naloxone.[70]

Nonopioid Analgesia in Amphibians

The AAT applied in studies using *Rana pipiens* clearly demonstrated dose-dependent and receptor-mediated opioid analgesia in amphibians. There were several other analgesic agents shown to be analgesic in typical rodent models that were also effective on the AAT. Potential nonopioid analgesics tested included antipsychotic, benzodiazepine, barbiturate, antihistamine, nonsteroidal anti-inflammatory drugs (NSAIDs), and partial opioid agents. Specifically, chlorpromazine and haloperidol (antipsychotics),

Table 1
Characteristics of opioid analgesics following systemic administration in *Rana pipiens*. The most potent drugs are listed first and in order of their calculated ED$_{50}$ values.

Opioid Agonist	Receptor Type	Dosage Range[a] (nmol/g)	ED$_{50}$ value[b] (nmol/g)	ED$_{50}$ value[c] (µg/g)
Fentanyl	mu	1–30	1.4	0.8
Enadoline	kappa	1–30	5.8	2.3
Remifentanil	mu	1–30	7.1	2.8
Levorphanol	mu	1–100	7.5	1.9
U50488H	kappa	1–100	8.5	3.1
Methadone	mu	10–300	19.9	6.2
Bremazocine	kappa	10–100	44.4	14.0
Morphine	mu	10–300	86.3	32.7
Buprenorphine	mu	30–300	99.1	46.3
Meperidine	mu	30–1000	128.1	31.6
Codeine	mu	10–1000	140.3	42.0
Nalorphine	kappa	100–300	320.9	99.9

[a] Effective dosage range in nmol/g body weight.
[b] Dose that gives 50% analgesic effects, in nmol/g body weight.
[c] Equivalent ED$_{50}$ in µg/g body weight dosing.
Data from Refs. [64,67]

chlordiazepoxide (a benzodiazepine), buprenorphine (partial opioid agonist), and diphenhydramine (histamine antagonist) produced moderate to strong analgesic effects.[71] Indomethacin and ketorolac (NSAIDs), butorphanol (partial opioid agonist), and pentobarbital (barbiturate) produced weaker but still had significant analgesic effects. Peak analgesic effects for the highest, nonlethal doses of the potent agents showed a relative analgesic potency of morphine > chlorpromazine > chlordiaz-epoxide > buprenorphine > diphenhydramine > haloperidol. It should be noted, however, that full dose-response curves were not generated, thus ED_{50} values were not calculated.

Studies by Brenner and colleagues and Suckow's group also demonstrated the analgesic efficacy of α_2-adrenergic agonists, such as clonidine, dexmedotomidine, and xylazine, at specific adrenergic receptor sites.[27,57,58] An additional NSAID agent, flunixin meglumine, was also an effective analgesic after intracelomic injection in *Rana pipiens*.[27] In a model of anesthesia using adult bullfrogs (*Rana catesbeiana*), it was noted that responses to strong forcep pinching of the hindlimb remained intact in animals anesthetized with thiopental, suggesting that this barbiturate is not a high-potency analgesic agent in amphibians. **Table 2** provides a summary of the doses tested and maximum percent effect (MPE) for nonopioid and partial opioids in behavioral studies in *Rana pipiens* following systemic administration.

CLINICAL APPLICATIONS OF AMPHIBIAN ANALGESIA

The clinical judgment of the attending veterinarian will ultimately determine the appropriate instances when an analgesic agent should be administered in an amphibian species. Cases of trauma to limbs or surgical interventions are possible scenarios when analgesics would be given. As pointed out in a recent opinion paper, the use

Table 2
Characteristics of nonopioid and partial opioid drugs following systemic administration in *Rana pipiens*

Agent	Class	Tested Dose[a] (nmol/g)	MPE[b]	Equivalent (µg/g)
Morphine	Opioid analgesic	300	100	114
Dexmedetomidine	α_2-Adrenergic	3	78.0	0.6
Chlorpromazine	Antipsychotic	100	62.9	32
Chlordiazepoxide	Benzodiazepine	300	51.3	90
Buprenorphine	Partial opioid agonist	30	48.6	14
Clonidine	α_2-Adrenergic	300	45.0	69
Diphenhydramine	H1 antagonist	200	43.2	51
Haloperidol	Antipsychotic	30	41.1	11
Indomethacin	NSAID	300	39.6	107
Ketorolac	NSAID	100	39.1	26
Butorphanol	Partial opioid agonist	100	36.9	33
Pentobarbital	Barbiturate	30	27.7	8

Morphine is included for comparison. The most efficacious drugs are listed first and drugs producing less than 40% effect (MPE) are listed in Italic.
[a] nmol/mg. The conversion of nmol/mg body weight doses to µg/g body weight doses is given in the last column.
[b] MPE = maximum percent effect of analgesia observed at that dose in an average of 4–8 animals.
Data from Refs. [57,71]

the postoperative analgesics in African clawed frogs (Xenopus laevis) after surgery for removal of oocytes used in biomedical research is currently an unresolved clinical issue.[72] Frog oocytes are often used for electrophysiological and molecular pharmacology studies because of their large size and ability to express transfected mRNA into receptor or channel proteins. There are established guidelines now for many university researchers on oocyte harvesting by repeated laparotomy (cf Google search for "oocyte harvesting guidelines"). Most institutions copy the guidelines from the National Institutes of Health-Office of Animal Care and Use (NIH-OACU) in their most recent revision.[73] These NIH guidelines do not mention any use of analgesics for postoperative care, but do suggest that animals be monitored daily for "appetite as well as for any complications such as dehiscence or infection. Such adverse effects would be reasons for immediate euthanasia."

A minority of other institutional animal care and use committees (IACUC) guidelines for oocyte harvesting from Xenopus do explicitly state that analgesics should be given and provide doses, as in this example from the University of North Carolina: "Postoperative care should be provided as with any species. Suggested analgesics for Xenopus are butorphanol, 25 mg/kg intracelomic, or xylazine, 10 mg/kg intracelomic. Both butorphanol and xylazine have a calming effect." Other sets of guidelines, as in this example from the University of Buffalo-SUNY, are even more explicit and state outright that analgesia should be addressed: "All frogs should receive at least one dose of postoperative analgesia. Acceptable analgesics include: flunixin meglumine (25 mg/kg intracelomic once) and xylazine 10 mg/kg intracelomic, every 12–24 h." Both of these institutions are recommending agents and doses based on the single study by Terril-Robb and colleagues.[27] Further studies are needed to determine the relative potency of other opioid and nonopioid analgesics shown to be active in preclinical studies (see **Tables 1** and **2**).

The issue of hypothermia for amphibian anesthesia or analgesia is also inadequately addressed in scientific studies. The guidelines mentioned here for oocyte removal all state that hypothermia is not an adequate method for inducing analgesia or for performing surgical procedures. There was one elegant study that examined hypothermia-induced analgesia in Rana pipiens using the AAT.[74] These investigators found that placement of a tourniqueted limb in icewater did produce analgesia in the acetic acid test as compared with the untreated contralateral limb. Furthermore, this analgesic effect was blocked by administration of the general opioid antagonist, naltrexone, suggesting the involvement of endogenous opioid peptide release. This finding has to be interpreted in light of other studies showing that: (1) amphibians in cold-adaptation show a decrease in pain thresholds[75,76] and (2) amphibians that are immobilized or in stressful situations produce opioid-mediated stress analgesia.[54,77]

A major concern is the risk-benefit ratio of using experimental drugs on zoologic companion animals such as amphibians. Most clinical treatments in nonmammalian species are by definition experimental, as little research has or is being done using these earlier-evolved vertebrates. The use of clinical analgesics in amphibians should be undertaken by those veterinarians who are willing to explore the nonmammalian "pain" literature and come to their own evidence-based conclusions. Practical recommendations for amphibian analgesia should follow the edict "first do no harm."

SUMMARY

Preclinical and clinical studies of analgesia in amphibians are extremely limited. Almost all preclinical studies were done using Rana pipiens and the AAT, while the greatest clinical need is for treatment of Xenopus laevis with postoperative analgesics after harvesting of oocytes in academic research settings.[72] There are also several zoos and herpetological collections that may also benefit from clinical information in recognizing and treating potential pain states in amphibians. Besides the inherent need of pain and analgesia studies in amphibians to guide the clinical treatment of these zoologic companion animals, preclinical research using nonmammalian models has yielded a surprising wealth of information on the vertebrate evolution of endogenous opioid peptides[78–80] and opioid receptor systems.[81–84] There is a great need for further research that can be realized by increased awareness and funding of amphibian models by alternative animal model foundations, increased preclinical and clinical research using *Xenopus* species, and increased involvement of exotic companion animal veterinarians in the research process.

REFERENCES

1. Stevens CW. Alternatives to the use of mammals for pain research. Life Sci 1992; 50:901–12.
2. Stevens CW. An amphibian model for pain research. Lab Anim 1995;24:32–6.
3. Stevens CW. An alternative model for testing opioid analgesics and pain research using amphibians. In: van Zutphen LF, Balls M, editors. Animal alternatives, welfare and ethics. Amsterdam: Elsevier; 1997. p. 247–51.
4. Rose JD. The neurobehavioral nature of fishes and the question of awareness and pain. Rev Fish Sci 2002;10:1–38.
5. Downes H, Koop DR, Klopfenstein B, et al. Retention of nociceptor responses during deep barbiturate anesthesia in frogs. Comp Biochem Physiol 1999;124:203–10.
6. Lafortune M, Mitchell MA, Smith JA. Evaluation of medetomidine, clove oil and propofol for anesthesia of leopard frogs, *Rana pipiens*. J Herpetol Med Surg 2001;11:13–8.
7. Barter LS, Antognini JF. Kinetics and potency of halothane, isoflurane, and desflurane in the northern leopard frog *Rana pipiens*. Vet Res Commun 2008;32: 357–65.
8. Guénette SA, Hélie P, Beaudry F, et al. Eugenol for anesthesia of African clawed frogs (*Xenopus laevis*). Vet Anesth Analgesia 2007;34:164–70.
9. Guénette SA, Beaudry F, Vachon P. Anesthetic properties of propofol in African clawed frogs (*Xenopus laevis*). J Am Assoc Lab Anim Sci 2008;47:35–8.
10. Stevens CW. Opioid antinociception in amphibians. Brain Res Bull 1988;21: 959–62.
11. Stevens CW. Non-mammalian models for the study of pain. In: Conn PM, editor. Sourcebook of models for biomedical research. Totowa (NJ): Humana Press; 2008. p. 341–52.
12. Greenacre C, Paul-Murphy J, Sladky KK, et al. Reptile and amphibian analgesia. J Herpetol Med Surg 2005;15:24–30.
13. Paul-Murphy J, Ludders JW, Robertson SA, et al. The need for a cross-species approach to the study of pain in animals. J Am Vet Med Assoc 2004;224:692–7.
14. Stevens CW. Alternative models for pain research: a translational, non-mammalian model with an ethical advantage. In: Warnick JE, Kalueff AV, editors. Translational neuroscience in animal research: advancement, challenges, and research ethics. Hauppauge (NY): Nova Science; 2010. p. 3–27.
15. Beer C. Motives and metaphors in considerations of animal nature. In: Pfaff DW, editor. Considerations of animal nature. New York: Springer-Verlag; 1983. p. 125–51.
16. Stevens CW. Opioid research in amphibians: an alternative pain model yielding insights on the evolution of opioid receptors. Brain Res Rev 2004;46:204–15.

17. Adrian ED, Cattell M, Hoagland H. Sensory discharges in single cutaneous nerve fibres. J Physiol 1931;72:377–91.
18. Maruhashi J, Mizuguchi K, Tasaki I. Action currents in single afferent nerve fibres elicited by stimulation of the skin of the toad and the cat. J Physiol 1952;117: 129–51.
19. Hamamoto DT, Simone DA. Characterization of cutaneous primary afferent fibers excited by acetic acid in a model of nociception in frogs. J Neurophysiol 2003;90: 566–77.
20. Nikundiwe AM, De Boer-van Huizen R, Ten Donkelaar HJ. Dorsal root projections in the clawed toad (*Xenopus laevis*) as demonstrated by anterograde labeling with horseradish peroxidase. Neuroscience 1982;7:2089–103.
21. Joseph BS, Whitlock DG. The morphology of spinal afferent-efferent relationships in vertebrates. Brain Behav Evol 1968;1:2–18.
22. Lorez HP, Kemali M. Substance P, met-enkephalin and somatostatin-like immunoreactivity distribution in the frog spinal cord. Neurosci Lett 1981;26:119–24.
23. Inagaki S, Senba E, Shiosaka S, et al. Regional distribution of substance P-like immunoreactivity in the frog brain and spinal cord: immunohistochemical analysis. J Comp Neurol 1981;201:243–54.
24. Yaksh TL, Stevens CW. Properties of the modulation of spinal nociceptive transmission by receptor-selective agents. In: Dubner R, Gebhart GF, Bond MR, editors. Proceedings of the 5th world congress on pain. Amsterdam: Elsevier; 1988. p. 417–35.
25. Simpson JI. Functional synaptology of the spinal cord. In: Llinas R, Precht W, editors. Frog neurobiology: a handbook. Berlin: Springer-Verlag; 1976. p. 728–49.
26. Rothe-Skinner KS, Stevens CW. Distribution of opioid-expressing neurons in the frog: an in situ hybridization study. Analgesia 1995;1:683–6.
27. Terril-Robb L, Suckow M, Grigdesby C. Evaluation of the analgesic effects of butorphanol tartrate, xylazine hydrochloride, and flunixin meglumine in leopard frogs (*Rana pipiens*). Contemp Top Lab Anim Sci 1996;35:54–6.
28. Machin KL. Fish, amphibian, and reptile analgesia. Vet Clin North Am Exot Anim Pract 2001;4:19–33.
29. Machin KL. Amphibian pain and analgesia. J Zoo Wildl Med 1999;30:2–10.
30. Verhaert P, De Loof A. Immunocytochemical localization of a methionine-enkephalin-resembling neuropeptide in the central nervous system of the American cockroach, *Periplaneta americana* L. J Comp Neurol 1985;239:54–61.
31. Hanke J, Jaros PP, Willig A. Autoradiographic localization of opioid binding sites combined with immunogold detection of Leu-enkephalin, crustacean hyperglycaemic hormone and moult inhibiting hormone at the electron microscopic level in the sinus gland of the shore crab, *Carcinus maenas*. Histochemistry 1993;99: 405–10.
32. Kavaliers M, Hirst M, Teskey GC. A functional role for an opiate system in snail thermal behavior. Science 1983;220:99–101.
33. Hanke J, Willig A, Jaros PP. Opioid receptor types for endogenous enkephalin in the thoracic ganglion of the crab, *Carcinus maenas*. Peptides 1996;17:965–72.
34. Spray DC. Cutaneous receptors: pain and temperature receptors of anurans. In: Llinas R, Precht W, editors. Frog neurobiology: a handbook. Berlin: Springer-Verlag; 1976. p. 607–28.
35. Vesselkin NP, Agayan AL, Nomokonova LM. A study of thalamo-telencephalic afferent systems in frogs. Brain Behav Evol 1971;4:295–306.
36. Munoz A, Munoz M, Gonzalez A, et al. Spinal ascending pathways in amphibians: cells of origin and main targets. J Comp Neurol 1997;378:205–28.

37. White JC, Sweet WH. Pain and the neurosurgeon. Springfield (IL): Thomas; 1969.
38. Talbot JD, Marrett S, Evans AC, et al. Multiple representations of pain in human cerebral cortex. Science 1991;251:1355–8.
39. Andrews EJ, Bennett BT, Clark JD, et al. 1993 report of the AVMA panel on euthanasia. J Am Vet Med Assoc 1993;202:229–49.
40. Smith JA, Boyd KM. Lives in the balance. Oxford (UK): Oxford University Press; 1991. p. 1–295.
41. Van Sluyters RC. Handbook for the use of animals in neuroscience research. Washington, DC: Society for Neuroscience; 1991.
42. Bardo MT, Hughes RA. Exposure to a nonfunctional hot plate as a factor in the assessment of morphine-induced analgesia and analgesic tolerance in rats. Pharmacol Biochem Behav 1978;10:481–5.
43. Pezalla PD. Morphine-induced analgesia and explosive motor behavior in an amphibian. Brain Res 1983;273:297–305.
44. Fukson OI, Berkinblit MB, Feldman AG. The spinal frog takes into account the scheme of its body during the wiping reflex. Science 1980;209:1261–3.
45. Hamamoto DT, Forkey MW, Davis WL, et al. The role of pH and osmolarity in evoking the acetic acid-induced wiping response in a model of nociception in frogs. Brain Res 2000;862:217–29.
46. Giszter SF, McIntyre J, Bizzi E. Kinematic strategies and sensorimotor transformations in the wiping movements of frogs. J Neurophysiol 1989;62:750–67.
47. Pezalla PD, Stevens CW. Behavioral effects of morphine, levorphanol, dextrophan and naloxone in the frog, Rana pipiens. Pharmacol Biochem Behav 1984;21:213–7.
48. Stevens CW, Pezalla PD. A spinal site mediates opiate analgesia in frogs. Life Sci 1983;33:2097–103.
49. Stevens CW, Pezalla PD. Naloxone blocks the analgesic action of levorphanol but not of dextrophan in the leopard frog. Brain Res 1984;301:171–4.
50. Stevens CW, Pezalla PD, Yaksh TL. Spinal antinociceptive action of three representative opioid peptides in frogs. Brain Res 1987;402:201–3.
51. Stevens CW, Toth G, Borsodi A, et al. Xendorphin B1, a novel opioid-like peptide determined from a Xenopus laevis brain cDNA library, produces opioid antinociception after spinal administration in amphibians. Brain Res Bull 2007;71:628–32.
52. Stevens CW, Martin KK, Stahlheber BW. Nociceptin produces antinociception after spinal administration in amphibians. Pharmacol Biochem Behav 2008;91:436–40.
53. Stevens CW, Kirkendall K. Time course and magnitude of tolerance to the analgesic effects of systemic morphine in amphibians. Life Sci 1993;52:PL111–6.
54. Stevens CW, Sangha S, Ogg BG. Analgesia produced by immobilization stress and an enkephalinase-inhibitor in amphibians. Pharmacol Biochem Behav 1995;51:675–80.
55. Willenbring S, Stevens CW. Thermal, mechanical and chemical peripheral sensation in amphibians: opioid and adrenergic effects. Life Sci 1996;58:125–33.
56. Willenbring S, Stevens CW. Spinal mu, delta and kappa opioids alter chemical, mechanical and thermal sensitivities in amphibians. Life Sci 1997;61:2167–76.
57. Brenner GM, Klopp AJ, Deason LL, et al. Analgesic potency of alpha-adrenergic agents after systemic administration in amphibians. J Pharmacol Exp Ther 1994;270:540–5.
58. Stevens CW, Brenner GM. Spinal administration of adrenergic agents produces analgesia in amphibians. Eur J Pharmacol 1996;316:205–10.

59. Newman LC, Wallace DR, Stevens CW. Characterization of 3H-diprenorphine binding in *Rana pipiens*: observations of filter binding enhanced by naltrexone. J Pharmacol Toxicol Methods 1999;41:43–8.
60. Stevens CW, Newman LC. Spinal administration of selective opioid antagonists in amphibians: evidence for an opioid unireceptor. Life Sci 1999;64:PL125–30.
61. Newman LC, Wallace DR, Stevens CW. Selective opioid agonist and antagonist displacement of [^{3}H]-naloxone binding in amphibian brain. Eur J Pharmacol 2000;397:255–62.
62. Newman LC, Wallace DR, Stevens CW. Selective opioid receptor agonist and antagonist displacement of [^{3}H]-naloxone binding in amphibian spinal cord. Brain Res 2000;884:184–91.
63. Newman LC, Sands SS, Wallace DR, et al. Characterization of mu, kappa, and delta opioid binding in amphibian whole brain tissue homogenates. J Pharmacol Exp Ther 2002;301:364–70.
64. Stevens CW, Klopp AJ, Facello JA. Analgesic potency of mu and kappa opioids after systemic administration in amphibians. J Pharmacol Exp Ther 1994;269:1086–93.
65. Stevens CW. Relative analgesic potency of mu, delta and kappa opioids after spinal administration in amphibians. J Pharmacol Exp Ther 1996;276:440–8.
66. Stevens CW, Rothe KS. Supraspinal administration of opioids with selectivity for mu, kappa, and delta opioid receptors produces analgesia in amphibians. Eur J Pharmacol 1997;331:15–21.
67. Mohan S, Stevens CW. Systemic and spinal administration of the mu opioid, remifentanil, produces antinociception in amphibians. Eur J Pharmacol 2006;534:89–94.
68. Benyhe S, Hoffmann Gy, Varga E, et al. Effects of oxymorphazone in frogs: long lasting antinociception in vivo, and apparently irreversible binding in vitro. Life Sci 1989;44:1847–57.
69. Koeller CA. Comparison of buprenorphine and butorphanol analgesia in the eastern red-spotted newt (*Notophthalmus viridescens*). J Am Assoc Lab Anim Sci 2009;48:171–5.
70. Kanetoh T, Sugikawa T, Sasaki I, et al. Identification of a novel frog RFamide and its effect on the latency of the tail-flick response of the newt. Comp Biochem Physiol C Toxicol Pharmacol 2003;134:259–66.
71. Stevens CW, MacIver DN, Newman LC. Testing and comparison of non-opioid analgesics in amphibians. Contemp Top Lab Anim Sci 2001;40:23–7.
72. Green SL. Postoperative analgesics in South African clawed frogs (*Xenopus laevis*) after surgical harvest of oocytes. Comp Med 2003;53:244–7.
73. Wyatt R. Guidelines for egg and oocyte harvesting in *Xenopus laevis*. National Institutes of Health, Office of Animal Care and Use. Washington, DC; 2007.
74. Suckow M, Terril L, Grigdesby C, et al. Evaluation of hypothermia-induced analgesia and influence of opioid antagonists in leopard frogs (*Rana pipiens*). Pharmacol Biochem Behav 1999;63:39–43.
75. Stevens CW, Pezalla PD. Endogenous opioid system down-regulation during hibernation in amphibians. Brain Res 1989;494:227–31.
76. Stevens CW. Environmental factors influencing pain physiology in amphibians. In: Mallick BN, Singh R, editors. Environment and physiology: 38th annual conference of the association of physiologists and pharmacologists of India. New Delhi (India): Narosa Publishing House; 1994. p. 54–61.
77. Pezalla PD, Dicig M. Stress-induced analgesia in frogs: evidence for the involvement of an opioid system. Brain Res 1984;296:356–60.

78. Dores RM, Lecaude S, Bauer D, et al. Analyzing the evolution of the opioid/orphanin gene family. Mass Spectrom Rev 2002;21:220–43.
79. Dores RM, Lecaude S. Trends in the evolution of the proopiomelanocortin gene. Gen Comp Endocrinol 2005;142:81–93.
80. Alrubaian J, Lecaude S, Barba J, et al. Trends in the evolution of the preprodynorphin gene in teleosts: Cloning of eel and tilapia prodynorphin cDNAs. Peptides 2006;27:797–804.
81. Stevens CW. Opioid research in amphibians: a unique perspective on mechanisms of opioid analgesia and the evolution of opioid receptors. Rev Analg 2003;7:122–36.
82. Stevens CW, Brasel CM, Mohan S. Cloning and bioinformatics of amphibian mu, delta, kappa, and nociceptin opioid receptors expressed in brain tissue: evidence for opioid receptor divergence in mammals. Neurosci Lett 2007;419:189–94.
83. Stevens CW. The evolution of vertebrate opioid receptors. Front Biosci 2009;14:1247–69.
84. Brasel CM, Sawyer GW, Stevens CW. A pharmacological comparison of the cloned frog and human mu opioid receptors reveals differences in opioid affinity and function. Eur J Pharmacol 2008;599:36–43.

Pain and Nociception in Reptiles

Craig Mosley, DVM, MSc, DACVA

KEYWORDS

• Pain • Nociception • Analgesia • Reptile

CLINICAL APPROACHES TO ANALGESIA IN REPTILES

The analgesic management of reptiles is challenging because of their unique physiologic, anatomic, and behavioral adaptations. As the number of studies examining pain and nociception in reptiles increases, our ability to provide analgesic care improves. The terms pain and nociception are frequently used interchangeably; however, in animals it may be worth differentiating between the 2 terms. Pain is inherently subjective, and is defined as unpleasant sensory and emotional experience associated with actual or potential tissue damage, or described in terms of such damage, noting that the inability to communicate verbally does not negate the possibility that an individual is experiencing pain and is in need of appropriate pain-relieving treatment.[1] Nociception generally refers to the physiologic or neuroanatomical components necessary to sense and transmit the noxious stimuli to the brain where it can ultimately be interpreted as a painful experience (ie, pain). The neuroanatomic components necessary for nociception have been described in reptiles.[2,3] In addition, endogenous antinociceptive mechanisms[3,4] and a demonstrable modulation of nociception with pharmacologic agents known to be analgesics in other species have been established.[5–11] In Tokay gecko lizards (Gekko gecko), spinal projections originating in the brainstem region (nucleus raphes inferior) that project to the superficial layers of the dorsal horn have been identified, and these structures suggest the presence of tracts that mediate descending inhibition of nociception, similar to those found in mammals.[8] Neurotransmitters that are important in nociceptive modulation in mammals have been identified in reptiles.[12] Whereas endogenous opioids and opioid receptors involved in reproduction and thermoregulation have been identified in reptiles, there is little known about the role of opioids in nociception.[12–15] This information suggests that at least at the physiologic level reptiles are capable of responding to noxious stimuli in a manner similar to mammals. The ability of reptiles to "feel" pain and the significance of pain or nociception on physiologic homeostasis is an exceedingly complex question requiring integration of both physiologic and behavioral evidence. Until further information is

The author has nothing to disclose.

Department of Anesthesia, Canada West Veterinary Specialists, 1988 Kootenay Street, Vancouver, British Columbia V5M 4Y3, Canada

E-mail address: c.mosley96@yahoo.ca

Vet Clin Exot Anim 14 (2011) 45–60

doi:10.1016/j.cvex.2010.09.009

1094-9194/11/$ – see front matter © 2011 Elsevier Inc. All rights reserved.

vetexotic.theclinics.com

available, it would seem most ethical for veterinarians to assume that reptiles are capable of feeling pain and to treat or manage pain when there is reasonable evidence that pain is present. In a survey of the membership of the Association of Reptile and Amphibian Veterinarians, 98% of the respondents indicated their belief that reptiles feel pain. However, only 39% of respondents in this survey reported using analgesics in more than 50% or their patients.[16] The reasons for failure to use analgesics were not specifically addressed in this study, yet possibilities include a failure to recognize painful patients, lack of efficacy data, concern regarding adverse effects, and little or no experimentally determined dose or pharmacokinetic information. With increased information available regarding analgesic use in reptiles and with the heightened awareness of the importance of analgesia for zoologic companion animals, it is likely that more veterinarians will provide pain relief to their reptile patients.

The benefits of providing adequate analgesia are well recognized in mammals. The consequences of untreated pain lead to impaired physiologic homeostasis in animals. These alterations can result in negative energy balance, lead to immune system compromise, inhibit healing, and interfere with normal behavioral processes required for health.[17,18]

Preemptive analgesic techniques are also gaining recognition, leading to postoperative pain reduction and preventing and/or limiting the actions of detrimental neurohumoral responses to pain.[19,20] The use of analgesics as part of a balanced anesthetic protocol can reduce the doses of other anesthetics, which can help reduce the negative cardiopulmonary effects of general anesthesia. Overall it has been demonstrated in humans and other mammals that appropriate analgesia is an important part of complete medical care in health and disease.

ASSESSING PAIN IN REPTILES

Appropriate pain management in nonverbal species, including human infants, is an extremely challenging endeavor requiring valid and reliable assessment techniques. Adult humans can express their individual level of pain and its significance to them. In nonverbal humans and animals, behavioral assessment tends to be the best indicator of pain.[21–23] However, with more than 8000 different reptile species identified that exhibit a wide range of unique physiologic and behavioral adaptations, it is exceedingly difficult to assess behavior changes in these animals. This situation makes behavioral alterations associated with pain particularly difficult to identify in reptiles. Recognition of abnormal behavior in reptiles requires careful, often time-consuming observation, and changes may be very subtle. An approach similar to pain assessment in other veterinary species can be adapted for use in reptiles (**Box 1**). If possible, it is best to observe reptiles using a remote camera based on evidence that reptiles may suppress some pain behaviors when an observer is present.[26] This response may be a protective one, similar to that seen in some reptiles subjected to brief physical restraint,[5] and is likely a normal protective behavioral response to a perceived threat, similar to that found in other vertebrate species.[27] A survey of reptile veterinarians found that the anticipated level of pain extrapolated from other species (76%), behavioral changes (66%), anticipated level of pain based on prior experience in reptiles (57%), and physiologic changes (32%) were commonly used to evaluate pain in reptiles.[16]

CHALLENGES OF STUDYING "PAIN" IN REPTILES

Studying most biologic phenomena requires some clearly defined measure of outcome. Studying "pain" is no different except that "pain" is an exceedingly difficult outcome to quantify and define because there is no single gold standard method to quantify pain in veterinary patients or humans.[28] Pain implies an unpleasant sensory or emotional experience and is especially difficult to quantify in patients unable to use language to describe this emotional event, for example, nonverbal humans (ie, pediatrics) or other nonhuman animals. However, as mentioned previously, the inability to communicate does not mean an animal is incapable of feeling pain. Pain reporting in humans is a composite of an individual's interpretation of the nociceptive insult that leads to the painful experience, and is influenced by a myriad of factors (ie, emotional state, concurrent diseases, concurrent medications, prior experience, sex, social status, environmental and economic factors, and so forth).[29–33] It is therefore not uncommon for two individuals subjected to the exact same level of tissue injury to quantify their pain quite differently.[30,33] In veterinary medicine it is probably unrealistic to assume that we can quantify pain in our patients with exact precision, as many of the same factors influencing pain reporting in humans are present when we attempt to interpret pain in our patients.[34–37]

There are many pain scales and questionnaires that have been developed to capture and quantify the individual pain experience for verbal humans. Several of these scales and questionnaires have been rigorously validated and widely adopted for clinical and research use[38]; by contrast, in veterinary medicine we have very few well-validated pain scales. The lack of widely accepted and validated pain scales makes it difficult to interpret conclusions and compare results among animal pain studies.

Pain in animals is most often quantified using semiobjective pain scales. These pain scales are developed using a combination of behavioral and physiologic factors believed to be associated with pain, although most measurable physiologic factors have not been shown to correlate strongly with pain. Pain scales range from very simple visual analog scales (consisting of a line representing the range; no pain to worst pain imaginable) to more complex multivariable numerical ratings scales. Regardless of the specific scale used, all rely on the user to correctly identify pain-related behaviors and/or pain-related physiologic alterations in the patient. Unfortunately, most pain scales are quite context specific and only suitable for assessing a particular type of pain (ie, acute or chronic), and are frequently species specific. Pain scales in veterinary medicine are continually being refined, modified, and tested as our level of sophistication in recognizing and quantifying pain related behaviors improves.

Pain-related behaviors that are crucial for the study of pain and analgesia are not well recognized in reptiles and hence surrogate methods are often required to assess analgesic efficacy. Some techniques attempt to use indirect indicators of analgesia, such as a reduction of the inhalant requirements needed to perform surgery,[39] as evidence of an analgesic effect. However, this technique can be unreliable and should not be used alone to infer analgesic potency.[40]

Another technique commonly used is to measure the response to a noxious stimuli (mechanical, thermal, or chemical threshold testing) with and without a prospective analgesic drug. These responses are most commonly characterized as nocifensive behaviors and as such are believed to be functionally related to pain but not entirely equivalent. This type of testing has been used extensively in mammals for assessing pain and analgesia, and has been shown to correlate well with the clinical efficacy of many drugs.[41,42] However, the predictive validity of these tests with nonopioid drugs is imperfect, and many weaknesses in these models have been described.[42,43] Thermal threshold testing is probably the model most often used for assessing acute nociception in veterinary studies. This technique is nearly ideal, as the noxious stimulus (heat)

Box 1
An approach to pain assessment in reptiles

Behavior

Species Considerations

Requires proper species identification and familiarity with species-specific behaviors. Basic species differences will impact behavioral patterns and these will be important when attempting to differentiate normal from abnormal behaviors.

  Predominant activity pattern (diurnal, nocturnal)

  Predated or predator species

  Habitat (arboreal, aquatic, terrestrial, fossorial)

Individual Patient Considerations

  Stage of ecdysis

    Some may become more aggressive during this time

  Hibernation status

    Hibernating animals or those inclined to hibernate may be more docile and less responsive than normal

  Socialization

    Altered response to human interaction (ie, a normally docile animal biting or poor response to caregiver)

  Concurrent illness

    Patient may be incapable of exhibiting behaviors associated with pain or behaviors associated with disease may be mistaken for pain behaviors

  Owner assessment

    Owners are often more familiar with their animals normal behavior, however owners may also be biased based on their own understanding and belief regarding their animals conditions

Environmental Considerations

  Enclosure

    Home enclosures often more "complex," compared with hospital enclosures, providing animal with plenty of opportunity to exhibit normal behaviors

  Preferred optimal body temperature observer

    Ambient environmental temperature is one of the main determinants of metabolic rate in resting reptiles and consequently normal behavior may influenced by alterations in metabolic rate

Locomotor Activity

  Posture

    Hunched, guarding of affected body area, not resting in normal posture

  Gait

    Must differentiate neurologic and mechanical dysfunction from pain induced lameness

  Other

    Excessive scratching or flicking foot tail or affected area

    Unwillingness to perform normal movements (look up, step up, thrash with tail)

    Exaggerated flight response

Miscellaneous

Appetite

Reduced appetite may be related to underlying disease but may also be related to pain

Eyes

Species with eyelids may close lids when painful or ill

Color change

Species capable of color change may do so in response to stress and/or pain

Abnormal respiratory movements

May be associated with primary respiratory disease but also pain affecting the muscles and tissues involved in respiration

Anticipated Level of Pain

The anticipated level of pain is commonly used to evaluate pain in reptiles and is based on the likelihood and severity of tissue trauma associated with a particular procedure or condition. This is a well-accepted approach in veterinary medicine, particularly when dealing with less familiar species.[24,25] However, in addition to significant species differences, significant individual differences in response to therapy and response to tissue trauma can be seen

Physiologic Data

Most physiologic parameters have been shown to be relatively poor indicators of pain in most species. Physiologic parameters can be influenced by disease and excitement. In addition, the physiologic parameters of reptiles may be influenced by several metabolic processes such as activity level, temperature alterations, and feeding

Response to Palpation

In some species a negative response to palpation can be a useful indicator of pain. However, in reptiles this may be less sensitive as most reptiles will withdraw from touch regardless of whether the animal is experiencing pain

---

is readily applied and removed, the latency is easily quantifiable, the behavior is explicit (the animal either does or does not withdraw from the stimulus), and the animal can immediately escape the noxious stimuli.[44] Thermal threshold testing has been used frequently in reptiles to assess the efficacy of various opioids, with very intriguing results.[6,7,9–11,26] However, reptiles are ectothermic, and the use of thermal threshold testing as an index for analgesic efficacy in reptiles raises some interesting questions. For example, would thermal thresholds change between a warming versus a cooling period in reptiles? Why are thermal burns so prevalent among captive reptiles? Could the intrinsic "drive" to warm increase thermal latency independent of drug? Would reptiles adapted to extreme environments (ie, desert animals experiencing hot days and cold nights) be more tolerant of heat than species normally inhabiting more temperate environments? It is possible that thermal latency in reptiles is affected by their thermal status (cooling, warming) and natural environmental adaptations. As thermal threshold testing is used more frequently to assess analgesic responses in reptiles, the application and strength of this method in ectothermic animals will be better understood.

Reptiles, unlike other commonly studied domestic animals such as dogs and cats, are not a single species; rather, they collectively represent more than 8000 species belonging to 4 distinct Orders: Crocodilia (crocodiles, alligators, caimans), Sphenodonita (tuataras), Squamata (snakes, lizards), and Chelonia (turtles, tortoises). The diversity among this population of animals makes it very difficult to make broad generalized recommendations for the entire group. Even among the limited number of reptile studies performed using very similar experimental techniques, marked differences in anesthetic requirements[39,45] and analgesic efficacy[9,10] have been observed.

Despite the challenges inherent in studying pain in reptiles, familiarity with normal behaviors of our reptile patients, using a systematic approach to evaluating pain and through the thoughtful use of information obtained from scientific studies we can greatly improve the overall comfort of our patients experiencing nociception and pain.

ANALGESIC THERAPY IN REPTILES

A carefully designed analgesic plan should include the specific analgesic drugs, route of drug administration, steps to monitor patient response to therapy and to address the provision of ongoing supportive patient care. Significant pharmacokinetic and pharmacodynamic differences exist between reptiles and mammals, making the extrapolation of drug dosing difficult. When available, species-specific analgesic drug studies in reptiles provide valuable insight to help guide analgesic therapy. However, critical evaluation is required to accurately interpret the results of these studies.

ROUTE OF DRUG ADMINISTRATION

The route of drug administration is an important consideration in reptiles for many reasons, including ease of administration, unique anatomic or physiologic structures, and variability in drug bioavailability and uptake among the various routes of drug administration.

Intravenous drug administration is the most predictable method for delivering a drug systemically. Intravascular injection ensures complete bioavailability of a drug and may avoid the tissue irritation associated with some drugs when given intramuscularly or orally. However, intravenous drug administration is not always feasible in reptiles but the combination of good technique, practice, appropriate patient selection, and skilled physical restraint can facilitate predictable venous access.

Intramuscular drug administration is a more convenient route for drug administration than the intravenous route but may be associated with reduced bioavailability. A study using green iguanas (*Iguana iguana*) found the bioavailability of ketoprofen when administered intramuscularly was 78%, representing a 28% reduction in bioavailability.[46] Historically, drug administration into the hind limb and tail has been avoided because of concerns about renal first-pass effect and renal toxicity associated with venous drainage into the renal portal system. In some species, this may be more of a theoretical than practical concern, as only a small amount of blood from the hind limbs and tail passes through the kidney,[47,48] whereas in other species a small amount from the hind limbs passes through the renal portal system while substantial amounts of blood from the tail passes through the renal portal system.[49] Therefore it may be best to avoid hind limb and tail administration of potentially nephrotoxic drugs or those highly metabolized or excreted by the kidneys, such as nonsteroidal anti-inflammatory drugs (NSAIDs). Another important consideration, less often discussed, is the possibility of a significant hepatic first-pass effect following hind limb drug administration. Anatomic studies performed in red-eared sliders showed that the femoral veins drained directly into the liver via the abdominal vein, creating ideal circumstances for significant presystemic hepatic extraction of drugs consequently leading to reduced drug bioavailability.[48] This hypothesis is supported by a recent study reporting approximately 70% relative bioavailability of buprenorphine injected into the hind limb versus the forelimb.[50] This finding is an important one because most opioids are susceptible to significant hepatic extraction,[51] further supporting the recommendation to preferentially use the forelimbs for drug administration.

Oral drug administration may be more desirable for patients who require chronic analgesic therapy, as most reptiles will become intolerant of repeated intramuscular injections. Oral drug administration can be difficult in some reptile patients, although the use of feeding tubes can markedly simplify and facilitate this process. An important consideration is the significant differences in gastrointestinal function among reptile species. Many are strict carnivores (snakes) and may fast for days to months between meals, whereas others are primarily herbivores (turtles, tortoises, and some lizards) and tend to feed more or less continuously. These differences would presumably affect the bioavailability and pharmacokinetics of drugs given orally among the different reptile species. However, a study in green iguanas found that the bioavailability and pharmacokinetics of meloxicam given orally was essentially the same as intravenous administration.[52]

DRUGS

There are 3 primary classes of analgesic drugs used in reptiles: opioids, local anesthetics, and NSAIDs (**Table 1**).

Opioids

It is well documented that reptiles have opioid receptors in the central nervous system[12,13] and that the proopiomelanocortin system (1 of the 3 molecular systems from which all naturally occurring opioids are derived) is well preserved among vertebrates.[63,64] The importance of the different opioid receptors in modifying nociception is far less clear and although increasing numbers of studies examining the role of opioids in reptile nociception are becoming available, each study should be carefully evaluated for the quality of experimental design and strength of its conclusions. Not surprisingly, the results of these studies suggest that the role of various opioid receptor agonists may vary among the reptile orders and even among species.

Butorphanol is a kappa-opioid receptor (KOR) agonist and mu-opioid receptor (MOR) antagonist, and is generally considered to be a mild analgesic in most veterinary species.[51] Similarly in reptiles, butorphanol, despite its frequent use,[16] does not appear to produce evidence of significant antinociceptive effects in all reptiles.[9,10,26,39,65] However, some studies suggest that certain doses of butorphanol in certain species may provide antinociception.[10,53] In one study, the intensity of motor reactions in response to an electrical stimulus applied to the tails of green iguanas was reduced.[53] However, the intensity of motor reactions was a subjectively evaluated parameter and may confound results. In another study, butorphanol administered at exceedingly high clinical doses (20 mg/kg intramuscularly) appeared to possess thermal antinociceptive properties in corn snakes, whereas using the same experimental model it failed to produce evidence of antinociception in bearded dragons (*Pogona vitticeps*)[10] and red-eared sliders (*Trachemys scripta elegans*).[9] Finally, in an experimental model using specific opioid receptor agonists, a pure KOR agonist failed to produce evidence of thermal antinociception in red-eared slider turtles.[11] Based on the accumulated data to date concerning butorphanol and its antinociceptive effects in reptiles it would seem that, at best, butorphanol may produce some antinociceptive effects at very high doses and that its clinical efficacy is highly questionable.

Table 1
Dosages of drugs with potential analgesic effects in reptiles

Drug	Dose (mg/kg)	Route	Interval (hours)	References	Comments
Opioids					
Butorphanol[a]	1.0–2.0	IM	NA	9,10,39,53,54	May not be effective as an analgesic in reptiles even at excessive doses
Buprenorphine	0.005–0.02 0.075–0.1	IM, IV, SC	NA	50,53,54	Analgesic effect not clearly demonstrated Pharmacokinetics have been determined in red-eared sliders Evidence of enterohepatic recycling
Morphine	0.05–4.0 (crocodiles) 1.5–6.5 (turtles) 1.0 (green iguanas)	IC, IM	NA	5,7,9,10,53,54	May require several hours to reach peak effect Duration of action may persist up to 24 h in turtles Significant respiratory depression in turtles
Meperidine	1.0–5.0	IC	NA	7,54,55	
Tramadol	10–25 10	PO SC	NA	56	Oral dose increased thermal nociceptive latency between 6 and 96 h SC dosing increased thermal nociception latency between 12 and 48 h Less respiratory depression than that from morphine

NSAIDs					
Carprofen[a]	1.0-4.0 followed by 1.0-2.0	IM, IV, SC	24-72[b]	54,55	
Flunixin meglumine[a]	0.1-2.0	IM	24-48[b]	54	
Ketoprofen	2.0	IM, SC	24-48[b]	46,54,55	PK determined for IM and IV administration
Meloxicam	0.1-0.2	IM, IV, PO	24-48[b]	52,54	PK determined for oral and intravenous administration in green iguanas. Evidence of enterohepatic recycling
Other					
Ketamine	<10	IM, IV, SC	NA	54	Low doses <10 mg/kg likely associated with analgesia without sedation
Medetomidine	50-100 μg/kg (tortoises); 150-300 μg/kg (aquatic); 150 μg/kg (snakes and lizards)	IM, IV, IO	NA	54,57-61	Lower doses may be effective for analgesia
Xylazine[a]	1-1.25	IM	NA	54	
Bupivacaine (0.5% or 0.25%)[a]	Toxic dose unknown, recommend <2 mg/kg	Local infiltration	NA	54,62	Dilute to 0.125% to increase volume
Lidocaine (2% or 1%)[a]	Toxic dose unknown, recommend <5 mg/kg	Local infiltration	NA	54,55	Dilute to 0.5% to increase volume

Abbreviations: IC, intracutaneous; IM, intramuscular; IV, intravenous; NA, interval dosing data unavailable, based on duration of clinical effect; PO, by mouth; SC, subcutaneous.

[a] Doses not determined experimentally, extrapolated or anecdotal.
[b] Dosing interval based on extrapolation.

Buprenorphine is a semisynthetic partial MOR agonist opioid with unique binding characteristics leading to a delayed onset and a long duration of action in mammals.[51] In the green iguana, buprenorphine did not significantly alter motor reactivity in response to an electrical stimulus when compared with saline.[53] However, these results may be unreliable owing to methodological limitations of the model and the markedly slower onset of action of buprenorphine compared with other opioids. The pharmacokinetics of buprenorphine have been determined in red-eared sliders and based on the results, a dosage of 0.075 to 0.1 mg/kg given subcutaneously in the fore-limb would maintain plasma drug concentrations at levels associated with analgesia in humans for at least 24 hours in 90% of red-eared sliders.[50] Of note, in the same study evidence of reduced buprenorphine bioavailability was evident when the drug was administered in the hind limb compared with the forelimb. The bioavailability of bupre-norphine following hind limb drug administration was 70% relative to forelimb drug administration. The reduced bioavailability was speculated to be the result of a hepatic first-pass extraction effect. The investigators also observed a secondary peak in plasma buprenorphine concentration occurring at around 72 hours following drug administration.[50] This secondary peak may be the result of enterohepatic recircula-tion, a phenomenon that has been detected in several other species.[66]

Morphine is a MOR agonist opioid with potent analgesic activity in most veterinary species and normally associated with minimal respiratory side effects when used at clinical doses.[51] However, the respiratory depression associated with MOR agonists can be exaggerated when combined with inhalant anesthetics and other sedatives.[51] There is considerable evidence that morphine may be effective as an analgesic in at least some reptile species.[6,7,9,10,53] It should be noted that time for onset of action appears to be prolonged (2–8 hours) following morphine administration, and the dura-tion of effect may vary considerably among species.[6,7,9,10] This process may be related to slow receptor-binding kinetics or slow absorption from the intramuscular or subcutaneous injection site.

Tramadol is an atypical synthetic opioid with weak MOR agonist activity and inhib-itory effects on neuronal reuptake of norepinephrine and serotonin.[51] Recent studies involving tramadol suggest it may be an effective long-lasting oral analgesic in reptiles. In red-eared sliders, tramadol administered orally (10–25 mg/kg) and parenterally (10 mg/kg) increased thermal nociceptive latency between 6 and 96 hours and 12 and 48 hours, respectively.[56]

Opioids appear to be safe for use in reptiles, even when relatively high doses are used, producing no discernible alterations in heart rate or behavior (sedation or excite-ment), but the MOR agonists (morphine) do cause significant respiratory depression in some species.[9,11,67,68] Conversely, opioids such as butorphanol and tramadol seem to be associated with less adverse respiratory effects.[9,11,56] In experimental studies with red-eared sliders using specific opioid receptor agonists, the respiratory depres-sant effects of opioids appeared to be mediated primarily via MOR and to a lesser extent via delta-opioid receptors (DOR).[69] However, the exact clinical significance of the respiratory depression described is not clear, as reptiles are well known to tolerate prolonged periods of hypoxia.[70–72] Nonetheless, it is prudent to support respi-ratory function in reptiles exhibiting profound respiratory depression.

Local Anesthetics

Local anesthetics act by interrupting transmission of sensory and motor neurons. In reptiles, local anesthetics are commonly used to facilitate minor surgical interventions but can also be used as local analgesics. Recently a technique has been described to block the mandibular nerve in crocodilians.[73] The limited duration of analgesic effect and accompanying motor paralysis associated with local anesthetics limit their use primarily to the immediate perioperative period or when hospitalized. Local anesthetic toxicity can be avoided by careful attention to total dose of local anesthetic administered to a patient. Many reptile patients are very small, and large doses can accidentally be administered. In general, the toxic doses of local anesthetics in mammals (dogs) should not be exceeded: lidocaine (toxic dose 10–22 mg/kg) and bupivacaine (toxic dose 5 mg/kg).[74] In addition, excessive dilution of local anesthetics may decrease their efficacy. To avoid reductions in efficacy, commercially available concentrations of local anesthetics should probably not be diluted more than 50%.[75,76] One percent lidocaine solution and 0.25% bupivacaine solutions are available commercially, and may be preferred for use in small patients at greater risk for local anesthetic toxicity.

NSAIDs

The role of cyclooxygenase in the pathophysiology of pain and inflammation of reptiles has not been studied. However, clinical reports support the efficacy of NSAIDs in reptiles, and they continue to be widely used.[16] There is only one study attempting to evaluate the analgesic efficacy of NSAIDs in reptiles, and the investigators found no decrease in the physiologic stress responses of ball pythons (Python regius) to surgery when meloxicam (0.3 mg/kg, intramuscular) was administered, suggesting it did not provide adequate analgesia.[65] However, it should be highlighted that even in the control animals given only saline there was little or no evidence to suggest that a stress response developed following their surgical procedure, and it was therefore difficult to assess whether meloxicam had an effect on diminishing the stress response.[65] The investigators acknowledge that the stress response was modest compared with that found after simply handling black racers (Coluber constrictor),[77] and although they make minimal comment, differences in technique could account for these discrepancies.

Meloxicam is probably the most widely used and recommended NSAID for reptiles. In pharmacokinetic studies, meloxicam administered orally to green iguanas had excellent bioavailability.[52] The results suggest that plasma concentrations associated with analgesia in other species are maintained in iguanas for 24 hours after a single oral dose of 0.2 mg/kg. Yet it should be noted that plasma concentrations of NSAIDs do not directly correspond to the clinical effect, and thus it is difficult to recommend effective and safe dosing intervals. There was also some evidence of enterohepatic or urinary resorption of meloxicam.[52] A pilot examination of the pharmacokinetics of ketoprofen administered intravenously and intramuscularly in green iguanas determined that bioavailability (78%) was decreased when administered intramuscularly and that terminal half-life was greater than in comparable studies in dogs.[46] This finding suggests that dosing intervals in reptiles should be longer than for mammals, a recommendation routinely followed for other drugs in reptiles, especially those associated with significant toxicity. Meloxicam administered daily at doses up to 5 mg/kg orally for 12 days produced no clinically apparent abnormalities or histopathological lesions associated with toxicity. However, mild biochemical and hematological abnormalities were noted that could not be clearly explained.[52] Another study involving daily administration of meloxicam and carprofen to green iguanas for 10 days similarly reported no clinical abnormalities but, did note some minor biochemical and hematological alterations that the investigators considered clinically insignificant.[78] Regardless of the apparent safety of NSAIDs in reptiles, it is advisable to consider the possibility that side effects similar to those seen in mammals (gastrointestinal [GI] irritation, renal compromise, platelet inhibition) may occur in reptiles. Therefore hydration status, concurrent medications such as steroids, presence of coagulopathy, GI disease, and renal disease should all be addressed before administering these drugs.

Other Drugs

Ketamine administered at subanesthetic doses is being used as an analgesic in many mammalian species, but its analgesic potential in reptiles has not been studied. Ketamine alone and used at anesthetic doses is associated with hypertension, tachycardia, bradypnea, and hypoventilation.[79–81] Ketamine may be a useful analgesic adjunct in select cases. The α_2 agonists produce analgesia, sedation, and muscle relaxation in mammals. In reptiles they appears to produce desirable levels of sedation and muscle relaxation. The analgesic effects of α_2 agonists have not been evaluated in reptiles but clinical impressions suggest they may be capable of producing an analgesic effect. Medetomidine induces cardiopulmonary effects in reptiles similar to those seen in mammals: bradycardia, hypertension, and a reduction in arterial oxygen partial pressures.[57,58] Other analgesic drugs and adjuncts such as tramadol, gabapentin, amantadine, the tricyclic antidepressants, various nutraceutical and physical therapy have not been explored in reptiles but may have a role to play as our understanding of nociception, pain, and analgesic therapy in reptiles increases.

SUMMARY

Reptiles are a very unique and diverse class of animals that have developed distinctive mechanisms, not found in most other animals, for managing alterations in body temperature and metabolic rate. An approach to pain management based on our current understanding of reptile physiology, nociception, pain, and analgesia represents a generalized approach to pain management in this class of animals. As our knowledge and understanding increases, it is likely that our approach to pain management in this class of animals will also be modified and refined to more specifically address reptile pain. New information should be evaluated objectively and without the influence of personal bias or beliefs. It is likely that reptiles have evolved unique mechanisms for managing pain and avoiding the negative consequences associated with pain that we do not yet completely understand.

REFERENCES

1. IASP. Part III: pain terms, a current list with definitions and notes on usage. In: Merskey H, Bogduk N, editors. Classification of chronic pain: descriptions of chronic pain syndromes and definitions of pain terms. 2nd edition. Seattle (WA): IASP Press; 1994. p. 209–14.
2. Liang YF, Terashima S. Physiological properties and morphological characteristics of cutaneous and mucosal mechanical nociceptive neurons with A-delta peripheral axons in the trigeminal ganglia of crotaline snakes. J Comp Neurol 1993;328:88.
3. Stoskopf MK. Pain and analgesia in birds, reptiles, amphibians, and fish. Invest Ophthalmol Vis Sci 1994;35:775.
4. Gans C, Gaunt AS. Muscle architecture and control demands. Brain Behav Evol 1992;40:70.
5. Mauk MD, Olson RD, LaHoste GJ, et al. Tonic immobility produces hyperalgesia and antagonizes morphine analgesia. Science 1981;213:353.
6. Kanui TI, Hole K, Miaron JO. Nociception in crocodiles: capsaicin instillation, formalin and hot plate tests. Zool Sci 1990;7:537.

7. Kanui TI, Hole K. Morphine and pethidine antinociception in the crocodile. J Vet Pharmacol Ther 1992;15:101.

8. ten Donkelaar HJ, de Boer-van HR. A possible pain control system in a non-mammalian vertebrate (a lizard, Gekko gecko). Neurosci Lett 1987;83:65.

9. Sladky KK, Miletic V, Paul-Murphy J, et al. Analgesic efficacy and respiratory effects of butorphanol and morphine in turtles. JAMA 2007;230:1356.

10. Sladky KK, Kinney ME, Johnson SM. Analgesic efficacy of butorphanol and morphine in bearded dragons and corn snakes. JAMA 2008;233:267.

11. Sladky KK, Kinney ME, Johnson SM. Effects of opioid receptor activation on thermal antinociception in red-eared slider turtles (*Trachemys scripta*). Am J Vet Res 2009; 70:1072.

12. de la Iglesia JA, Martinez-Guijarro FI, Lopez-Garcia C. Neurons of the medial cortex outer plexiform layer of the lizard *Podarcis hispanica*: golgi and immuno-cytochemical studies. J Comp Neurol 1994;341:184.

13. Reiner A. The distribution of proenkephalin-derived peptides in the central nervous system of turtles. J Comp Neurol 1987;259:65.

14. Lindberg I, White L. Reptilian enkephalins: implications for the evolution of proenkephalin. Arch Biochem Biophys 1986;245:1.

15. Ng TB, Hon WK, Cheng CH, et al. Evidence for the presence of adrenocortico-tropic and opiate-like hormones in the brains of two sea snakes, *Hydrophis cyanocinctus* and *Lapemis hardwickii*. Gen Comp Endocrinol 1986;63:31.

16. Read MR. Evaluation of the use of anesthesia and analgesia in reptiles. J Am Vet Med Assoc 2004;224:547.

17. Kona-Boun JJ, Silim A, Troncy E. Immunologic aspects of veterinary anesthesia and analgesia. J Am Vet Med Assoc 2005;226:355.

18. Muir WW. Pain and stress. In: Gaynor J, Muir WW, editors. Handbook of veterinary pain management. 2nd edition. Toronto: Mosby; 2009. p. 42.

19. Lascelles BD, Waterman AE, Cripps PJ, et al. Central sensitization as a result of surgical pain: investigation of the pre-emptive value of pethidine for ovariohysterectomy in the rat. Pain 1995;62:201.

20. Woolf CJ, Chong MS. Preemptive analgesia—treating postoperative pain by preventing the establishment of central sensitization. Anesth Analg 1993;77:362.

21. Holton L, Reid J, Scott EM, et al. Development of a behaviour-based scale to measure acute pain in dogs. Vet Rec 2001;148:525.

22. Pritchett LC, Ulibarri C, Roberts MC, et al. Identification of potential physiological and behavioral indicators of postoperative pain in horses after exploratory celiotomy for colic. Appl Anim Behav Sci 2003;80:31.

23. van Dijk M, de Boer JB, Koot HM, et al. The reliability and validity of the COMFORT scale as a postoperative pain instrument in 0 to 3-year-old infants. Pain 2000;84:367.

24. Flecknell PA. The relief of pain in laboratory animals. Lab Anim 1984;18:147.

25. Morton DB. Assessment of pain. Vet Rec 1986;119:435.

26. Fleming GJ, Robertson S. Use of thermal threshold test response to evaluate the antinociceptive effects of butorphanol in juvenile Green iguanas (Iguana iguana). In: American Association of Zoo Veterinarians. Tampa (FL); 2006. p. 279.

27. Porro CA, Carli G. Immobilization and restraint effects on pain reactions in animals. Pain 1988;32:289.

28. Mich PM, Hellyer PW. Objective, categoric methods for assessing pain and analgesia. In: Gaynor JS, Muir WW, editors. Handbook of veterinary pain management. 2nd edition. St. Louis (MO): Mosby Elsevier; 2009. p. 78.

29. Tsang A, Von Korff M, Lee S, et al. Common chronic pain conditions in developed and developing countries: gender and age differences and comorbidity with depression-anxiety disorders. J Pain 2008;9:883.

30. Fillingim RB. Individual differences in pain responses. Curr Rheumatol Rep 2005; 7:342.

31. Fillingim RB, King CD, Ribeiro-Dasilva MC, et al. Sex, gender, and pain: a review of recent clinical and experimental findings. J Pain 2009;10:447.

32. Nielsen CS, Stubhaug A, Price DD, et al. Individual differences in pain sensitivity: genetic and environmental contributions. Pain 2008;136:21.

33. Nielsen CS, Staud R, Price DD. Individual differences in pain sensitivity: measurement, causation, and consequences. J Pain 2009;10:231.

34. Hewson CJ, Dohoo IR, Lemke KA. Factors affecting the use of postincisional analgesics in dogs and cats by Canadian veterinarians in 2001. Can Vet J 2006;47:453.

35. Hewson CJ, Dohoo IR, Lemke KA. Perioperative use of analgesics in dogs and cats by Canadian veterinarians in 2001. Can Vet J 2006;47:352.

36. Hewson CJ, Dohoo IR, Lemke KA, et al. Factors affecting Canadian veterinarians' use of analgesics when dehorning beef and dairy calves. Can Vet J 2007;48: 1129.

37. Hewson CJ, Dohoo IR, Lemke KA, et al. Canadian veterinarians' use of analgesics in cattle, pigs, and horses in 2004 and 2005. Can Vet J 2007;48:155.

38. Melzack R, Katz J. Pain assessment in adult patients. In: McMahon SB, Koltzenburg M, editors. Wall and Melzack's textbook of pain. 5th edition. Philadelphia: Elsevier/Churchill Livingstone; 2005. p. 291.

39. Mosley CA, Dyson D, Smith DA. Minimum alveolar concentration of isoflurane in green iguanas and the effect of butorphanol on minimum alveolar concentration. J Am Vet Med Assoc 2003;222:1559.

40. Brosnan RJ, Pypendop BH, Siao KT, et al. Effects of remifentanil on measures of anesthetic immobility and analgesia in cats. Am J Vet Res 2009;70:1065.

41. Bennett GJ. Animal models in pain. In: Kruger L, editor. Methods in pain research. Boca Raton (FL): CRC Press, Inc; 2001. p. 67.

42. Le Bars D, Gozariu M, Cadden SW. Animal models of nociception. Pharmacol Rev 2001;53:597.

43. Negus SS, Vanderah TW, Brandt MR, et al. Preclinical assessment of candidate analgesic drugs: recent advances and future challenges. J Pharmacol Exp Ther 2006;319:507.

44. Hargreaves K, Dubner R, Brown F, et al. A new and sensitive method for measuring thermal nociception in cutaneous hyperalgesia. Pain 1988;32:77.

45. Bertelsen MF, Mosley CA, Crawshaw GJ, et al. Minimum alveolar concentration of isoflurane in mechanically ventilated dumeril monitors. J Am Vet Med Assoc 2005;226:1098.

46. Tuttle AD, Papich M, Lewbart GA, et al. Pharmacokinetics of ketoprofen in the green iguana (Iguana iguana) following single intravenous and intramuscular injections. J Zoo Wildl Med 2006;37:567.

47. Holz P, Barker IK, Burger JP, et al. The effect of the renal portal system on pharmacokinetic parameters in the red-eared slider (Trachemys scripta elegans). J Zoo Wildl Med 1997;28:386.

48. Holz P, Barker IK, Crawshaw GJ, et al. The anatomy and perfusion of the renal portal system in the red-eared slider (*Trachemys scripta elegans*). J Zoo Wildl Med 1997;28:378.

49. Benson KG, Forrest L. Characterization of the renal portal system of the common green iguana (Iguana iguana) by digital subtraction imaging. J Zoo Wildl Med 1999;30:235.

50. Kummrow MS, Tseng F, Hesse L, et al. Pharmacokinetics of buprenorphine after single-dose subcutaneous administration in red-eared sliders (*Trachemys scripta elegans*). J Zoo Wildl Med 2008;39:590.

51. Lamont LA, Mathews KA. Opioids, nonsteroidal anti-inflammatories, and analgesic adjuvants. In: Tranquilli WJ, Thurmon JC, Grimm KA, editors. Lumb and Jones' veterinary anesthesia and analgesia. 4th edition. Ames (IA): Blackwell Publishing; 2007. p. 241.

52. Hernandez-Divers SJ, McBride M, Koch T, et al. Single-dose oral and intravenous pharmacokinetics of meloxicam in the green iguana (*Iguana iguana*). Proc Assoc Rept Amphib Vet 2004;106.

53. Greenacre CB, Takle G, Schumacher J, et al. Comparative antinociception of morphine, butorphanol, and buprenorphine versus saline in the green iguana, *Iguana iguana*, using electrostimulation. J Herpetol Med Surg 2006;16:88.

54. Funk RS, Diethelm G. Reptile formulary. In: Mader DR, editor. Reptile medicine and surgery. 2nd edition. St. Louis (MO): Elsevier Inc; 2005. p. 1119.

55. Bennett RA. Reptile anesthesia. Seminars in Avian and Exotic Pet Medicine 1998; 7:30.

56. Cummings BB, Sladky KK, Johnson SM. Tramadol analgesic and respiratory effects in red-eared slider turtles (*Trachemys scripta*). In: American Association of Zoo Veterinarians and American Association of Wildlife Veterinarians Joint Conference. Tulsa (OK); 2009. p. 115.

57. Sleeman JM, Gaynor J. Sedative and cardiopulmonary effects of medetomidine and reversal with atipamezole in desert tortoises (*Gopherus agassizii*). J Zoo Wildl Med 2000;31:28.

58. Dennis PM, Heard DJ. Cardiopulmonary effects of a medetomidine-ketamine combination administered intravenously in gopher tortoises. J Am Vet Med Assoc 2002;220:1516.

59. Greer LL, Jenne KJ, Diggs HE. Medetomidine-ketamine anesthesia in red-eared slider turtles (*Trachemys scripta elegans*). Contemp Top Lab Anim Sci 2001;40:9.

60. Chittick EJ, Stamper MA, Beasley JF, et al. Medetomidine, ketamine, and sevoflurane for anesthesia of injured loggerhead sea turtles: 13 cases (1996–2000). J Am Vet Med Assoc 2002;221:1019.

61. Lock BA, Heard DJ, Dennis P. Preliminary evaluation of medetomidine/ketamine combinations for immobilization and reversal with atipamezole in three tortoise species. Bulletin of the Association of Reptilian and Amphibian Veterinarians 1998;8:6.

62. Redrobe S. Anaesthesia and analgesia. In: Girling S, Raiti P, editors. BSAVA manual of reptiles. Shurdington (Cheltenham): British Small Animal Veterinary Association; 2004. p. 131.

63. Zagon IS, Sassani JW, Allison G, et al. Conserved expression of the opioid growth factor, [Met5]enkephalin, and the zeta (zeta) opioid receptor in vertebrate cornea. Brain Res 1995;671:105.

64. Polzonetti-Magni A, Facchinetti F, Carnevali O, et al. Presence and steroidogenetic activity of beta-endorphin in the ovary of the lizard, Podarcis s. sicula raf. Biol Reprod 1994;50:1059.

65. Olesen MG, Bertelsen MF, Perry SF, et al. Effects of preoperative administration of butorphanol or meloxicam on physiologic responses to surgery in ball pythons. J Am Vet Med Assoc 2008;233:1883.

66. Brewster D, Humphrey MJ, McLeavy MA. Biliary excretion, metabolism and enterohepatic circulation of buprenorphine. Xenobiotica 1981;11:189.
67. Mosley CA, Dyson D, Smith DA. The cardiovascular dose-response effects of isoflurane alone and combined with butorphanol in the green iguana (*Iguana iguana*). Vet Anaesth Analg 2004;31:64.
68. Hinsch H, Gandal CP. The effects of etorphine (M-99), oxymorphone hydrochloride and meperidine hydrochloride in reptiles. Copeia 1969;404.
69. Johnson SM, Kinney ME, Wiegel LM. Inhibitory and excitatory effects of micro-, delta-, and kappa-opioid receptor activation on breathing in awake turtles, *Trachemys scripta*. Am J Physiol Regul Integr Comp Physiol 2008;295:R1599.
70. Bickler PE, Buck LT. Hypoxia tolerance in reptiles, amphibians, and fishes: life with variable oxygen availability. Annu Rev Physiol 2007;69:145.
71. Belkin DA. Anoxia: tolerance in reptiles. Science 1963;139:492.
72. Hochachka PW, Lutz PL. Mechanism, origin, and evolution of anoxia tolerance in animals. Comp Biochem Physiol B Biochem Mol Biol 2001;130:435.
73. Wellehan JF, Gunkel CI, Kledzik D, et al. Use of a nerve locator to facilitate administration of mandibular nerve blocks in crocodilians. J Zoo Wildl Med 2006;37:405.
74. Liu PL, Feldman HS, Giasi R, et al. Comparative CNS toxicity of lidocaine, etidocaine, bupivacaine, and tetracaine in awake dogs following rapid intravenous administration. Anesth Analg 1983;62:375.
75. Kanai A, Hoka S. A comparison of epidural blockade produced by plain 1% lidocaine and 1% lidocaine prepared by dilution of 2% lidocaine with the same volume of saline. Anesth Analg 2006;102:1851.
76. Kanai A, Koiso S, Hoka S. Comparison of analgesia induced by continuous epidural infusion of plain 1% lidocaine and 1% lidocaine prepared by dilution of 2% lidocaine with the same volume of saline. J Clin Anesth 2007;19:534.
77. Stinner JN, Ely DL. Blood pressure during routine activity, stress, and feeding in black racer snakes (Coluber constrictor). Am J Phys 1993;264:R79.
78. Trnkova S, Knotkova Z, Hrda A, et al. Effect of non-steroidal anti-inflammatory drugs on the blood profile in the green iguana (Iguana iguana). Vet Med 2007;52:507.
79. Arena PC, Richardson KC, Cullen LK. Anaesthesia in two species of large Australian skink. Vet Rec 1988;123:155.
80. Custer RS, Bush M. Physiologic and acid-base measures of gopher snakes during ketamine or halothane-nitrous oxide anesthesia. J Am Vet Med Assoc 1980;177:870.
81. Schumacher J, Lillywhite HB, Norman WM, et al. Effects of ketamine HCl on cardiopulmonary function in snakes. Copeia 1997;395.

Avian Analgesia

Michelle G. Hawkins, VMD, DABVP (Avian Practice)*,
Joanne Paul-Murphy, DVM, DACZM

KEYWORDS
- Analgesia • Pain • Bird • NSAID • Opioid

RECOGNIZING PAIN IN BIRDS

All vertebrate animals share similar neuroanatomic and neuropharmacologic components required for nociception, detection, transmission, and response to noxious stimuli. Pain is the sensory and emotional experience associated with actual or potential tissue damage. Pain affects the animal's physiology and behavior to reduce or avoid the damage, to reduce the likelihood of recurrence and to promote recovery. Assessment of pain must account for species, gender, age, strain, environment, and concurrent disease. The type of pain such as acute, chronic, somatic, visceral, clinical, or neuropathic also affects the behavior of the bird. Pain is subjective and the emotional component is difficult for us to translate because most avian species lack facial expression and do not share verbal language with humans. In humans, we accept that pain is what the patient says it is, but with birds, people's perceptions of the bird's behavior determines what is recognized as pain.

Species variability occurs because of differences in pain sensitivity, the conscious response to pain, and the physiologic response to analgesic therapy. Genetic variability with response to pain has been demonstrated at the individual level and in different strains of chickens.[1,2] Behavioral changes can be very cryptic and subtle but are often the earliest signs of pain detected by animal care staff or owners. Behavioral change does not manifest uniformly among different species of birds and observers must be familiar with the full range of normal behaviors for the species as well as the individual. It is important to observe birds at appropriate times for each species; for example, observing nocturnal species at night. Without knowing the range of normal behavior, an observer will find it extremely difficult to detect abnormal behavior, especially in prey species, which often only demonstrate cryptic and subtle changes. The outward behavior of a companion bird acclimated to handling does not accurately reflect the physiologic changes occurring with stress-related hormones, respiratory rate, or body temperature.[3,4] Therefore it can be inferred that a bird in pain may also mask physiologic changes associated with the pain.

Certain behaviors have evolved over thousands of years and have survival value; for example, immobility is a common behavior displayed by birds when being observed or

Department of Medicine and Epidemiology, School of Veterinary Medicine, University of California, Davis, 2108 Tupper Hall, Davis, CA 95616, USA
* Corresponding author.
E-mail address: mghawkins@ucdavis.edu

Vet Clin Exot Anim 14 (2011) 61–80
doi:10.1016/j.cvex.2010.09.011
1094-9194/11/$ – see front matter © 2011 Elsevier Inc. All rights reserved.

examined, making pain evaluation challenging.[5] In chickens, crouching immobility has been associated with prolonged pain, stress, and fear responses. When a noxious stimulus was applied to ulcerated buccal lesions, chickens remained motionless in a crouchlike stance with the head pulled into the body and had significantly fewer alert head movements.[6] Removal of feathers from chickens caused a progression of behavioral changes from an alert agitated response following the initial removal of feathers to periods of crouching immobility following successive removal.[7]

Feather grooming is an avian behavior that runs the full spectrum of change associated with pain, both acute and chronic. Grooming activity may decrease when a bird is painful, but conversely over-grooming and feather destructive behaviors have been associated with chronic pain. In a social species housed with a group, a painful bird frequently isolates itself from the others, may sleep apart from the rest of the flock, and mutual grooming is often decreased.[4] In some species a display of discomfort, illness, or weakness may gain support or protection from conspecifics, but similar behavior in another species may attract attention from predators, or lower its status in the flock's social order.[8] Increased grooming activities to themselves or other birds can be an intentional distraction. Studies using chickens with experimental arthritis demonstrated that shifting attention can reduce painful behaviors and potentially reduce peripheral inflammation.[9]

Treating avian pain is limited by the reliability of pain assessment, which remains highly subjective, and clinicians often need to rely on indirect measures of pain. Having an identified behavior or set of behaviors that correlate with pain provides a response that can be used to monitor analgesic therapy. It is difficult to state when a bird's condition is effectively treated if it cannot be measured before and after therapy. Nonetheless, having an identified behavior or set of behaviors that correlate with pain provides a means to monitor response to pain treatment. Pain scales and score sheets are increasingly being used to assess pain in animals, especially when specifically designed for a given species under well-defined conditions. Using pain scales requires understanding of normal and pain-related behaviors for the species and individual under study. Pain score sheets can help maximize the efficacy of pain scoring using behavioral analysis. Score sheet descriptions of behavior must be refined, and terms must be clearly defined to reduce observer bias and interobserver variability. Once such a system is implemented, well-trained non-veterinary staff can perform scoring. These pain scales take time and effort to design.

Pain is not just a yes/no response, it occurs along a gradient. In lieu of species-specific pain score sheets for birds, there is tremendous value in using a generic pain scale of 1 to 10 to evaluate a bird's pain and the response to treatment and recovery from a painful condition. In a study completed by one of the authors, pigeons were evaluated after orthopedic surgery using a detailed numeric rating scale plus a simple 1 to 10 pain scale and there was significant correlation between both methods (J. Paul-Murphy, personal communication, July 1, 2010). Effective analgesia is expected to show a marked, easily discernable change in posture or behaviors that will effect a reliable change in the subjective pain score. If no change in pain score occurs, then the drugs, dose, or frequency of administration need to be reevaluated for that individual patient.

EVALUATION OF ANALGESICS

It is difficult to define and recognize when birds feel pain, and it can be even more challenging to objectively determine whether a pain medication is effective in the avian patient. To determine the efficacy of an analgesic in any species, it is important to determine the pharmacokinetic (PK) and pharmacodynamic (PD) properties of the drug in that species. Integrating PK and PD data can also provide a basis for selecting clinically relevant dosing schedules for subsequent evaluation in disease models and clinical trials.[10] When the same dose produces different plasma concentrations in different species of birds, the variance is due to PK. When the same plasma concentration produces different responses in different species, the variance is due to PD. PK studies of analgesic drugs are insufficient to determine appropriate doses and dosing frequencies as plasma concentrations of opioids and nonsteroidal antiinflammatory drugs (NSAIDs) do not always correlate with delivery of analgesia. Plasma concentrations provide guidance for dosing frequencies, but it has been shown that duration of analgesic effect of a NSAID may be longer than predicted from plasma levels. The PK of analgesics vary considerably across all species that have been studied, so extrapolating clinical doses and dosing intervals from one species to another species is not appropriate. To date, very few PK studies have been published for analgesics in birds (**Tables 1** and **2**).

Anesthetic sparing studies provide an in vivo PD technique for objective evaluation by measuring the reduction in the amount of inhaled anesthetic capable of maintaining a minimal level of anesthesia following administration of the analgesic under investigation. This type of testing has been used in many species to evaluate analgesic drug properties, particularly opioids. Although this approach provides meaningful information, there are limitations because the anesthetic itself can be a confounding variable and when evaluating opioids it is difficult to assess whether an observed effect is an analgesic or a sedative response to the drug.

Assessing the inhibition of serum inflammatory markers may be useful for evaluating one aspect of NSAID analgesia, but serum concentrations of markers do not give a complete picture of the effect because many inflammatory markers are found at the site of inflammation rather than in serum. Acute inflammation models have been developed in many species by injecting irritating materials into tissues and measuring inflammatory factors in exudates for differences with and without the NSAID. Avian patients most commonly produce caseous exudates, making it difficult to collect and evaluate peripheral inflammatory markers for evaluation of NSAIDs. Inflammatory models are also used to create painful conditions with repeatable behaviors or weight bearing that can be quantified such as acute synovitis/arthritis models in chickens and parrots.[16,18,20,24,26,34] In one model the injection of urate microcrystals into the intertarsal joint caused acute inflammatory arthritis leading to measurable changes in weight bearing and lameness. A study with Amazon parrots differentiated significant improvement in weight bearing when birds were given butorphanol versus less improvement in the same birds given carprofen.[26] Evaluating the response of a bird to a painful stimulus, also termed noxious stimulus, with and without analgesics is used to determine efficacy when behavioral responses or thresholds can be measured. The noxious stimuli used in avian analgesia studies are variable but usually include withdrawal thresholds to thermal, electrical, or pressure stimuli. Experimental models have been developed in chickens and parrots but these models may not extrapolate to pain behaviors relevant to clinical pain. Therefore, the doses and dosing frequencies recommended in the published reports should always be critically evaluated case by case when clinically applied.

PREVENTIVE OR PREEMPTIVE ANALGESIA

Recent evidence suggests that surgical incision and other painful procedures in humans may induce prolonged changes in the central nervous system (CNS) that later

Table 1
Opioid analgesics evaluated in avian species by either pharmacokinetic (PK) or pharmacodynamic (PD) studies

Drug	Dosage (mg/kg, unless noted)	Route	Frequency	Species	Comments	Type of Study	References
Butorphanol	0.5	IM, IV (median ulnar v; medial metatarsal v)	Single injection	Red-tailed hawks Great-horned owls	$t_{1/2}$ IV, IM very short (approx. 1–2 h); significantly more rapid clearance and shorter $t_{1/2}$ when given IV medial metatarsal than IV median ulnar v	PK	11
	5	Oral	Single dose	Hispaniolan Amazon parrots	Oral bioavailability<10%; do not recommend this route of administration	PK	12
	2–5	IM	Single injection	Hispaniolan Amazon parrots	PK: low mean plasma concentrations at 2 h after injection PD: withdrawal thresholds to electrical stimuli reduced after 2 mg/kg IM	PK/PD	13
	1	IM	Single injection	Cockatoos African gray parrots Blue-fronted Amazon parrots	Isoflurane-sparing study showed significant reduction in isoflurane MAC in the cockatoos and African grays, but not Amazon parrots	PD	14,15
	1–2	IM	Single injection	African gray parrots	Electrical stimuli to assess withdrawal thresholds; more significant reduction of withdrawal response at 2 mg/kg	PD	16
	3–6	IM	Single injection	Hispaniolan Amazon parrots	Electrical stimuli to assess withdrawal thresholds; 3 and 6 mg/kg effective	PD	16
	2	IM	Single injection	Hispaniolan Amazon parrots	Safe and effective preemptive analgesia with sevoflurane anesthesia for endoscopy	PD	17

Drug	Dose	Route	Species	Notes	PK/PD	Ref
Fentanyl	0.02 0.2	IM SC	Single injection Cockatoos	PK: rapid absorption and elimination PD: withdrawal thresholds to electrical and thermal stimuli. 0.02 mg/kg did not affect either threshold; 0.2 mg/kg did affect both withdrawal thresholds but only some birds; hyperactivity in first 15–30 min	PK/PD	18
	0.15–0.50 µg/kg/min	IV	Constant-rate infusion Red-tailed hawks	Reduced isoflurane MAC 31%–55% in a dose-related manner, without significant effects on heart rate, blood pressure, $Paco_2$, or Pao_2	PD	19
	0.05–1.0	Intraarticular	Single injection Chickens	No significant effect on induced arthritis	PD	20
Buprenorphine	0.1	IM	Single injection African gray parrots	PK: may not achieve effective plasma concentrations at this dose PD: no change in withdrawal response to noxious stimuli	PK/PD	16,21
	0.25 0.5	IM	Single injection Domestic pigeons	Increased latency period for withdrawal from a noxious electrical stimulus of 2 h at 0.25 mg/kg and for 5 h for 0.5 mg/kg	PD	22
	0.05–1.0	Intraarticular	Single injection Chickens	No significant effect on induced arthritis	PD	20
Nalbuphine	12.5 25 50	IM	Single injection Hispaniolan Amazon parrots	PK: $t_{1/2}$ IM and IV less than 0.35 h; Excellent IM bioavailability PD: 12.5 mg/kg produced 3 h analgesia; higher doses did not increase analgesic time	PD	23

Abbreviations: CR, care report or case series; IM, intramuscularly; IV, intravenously; PD, pharmacodynamic; PK, pharmacokinetic; TOX, toxicity; $t_{1/2}$, half-life; v, vein.

Table 2
NSAIDs evaluated in avian species by either pharmacokinetic (PK), pharmacodynamic (PD) evaluations, toxicologic (TOX) or clinical studies

Drug	Dosage (mg/kg)	Route	Frequency (Every hour)	Species	Comments	Type of Study	References
Sodium salicylate	100–200	IM	Single injection	Chickens	Arthritis painful behaviors partially reduced 1 h after ASA treatment	PD	24
	25	IV	Single injection	Chickens, ostrich, ducks, turkeys, pigeons	Rapid clearance except long $t_{1/2}$ in pigeon	PK	25
Carprofen	30	IM	Single injection	Chickens	Arthritis painful behaviors reduced 1 h after treatment	PD	24
	3	IM	12	Hispaniolan Amazon parrots	Arthritis pain partially reduced, effect less than 12 h	PD	26
	1	IM	Single injection	Chickens	Improved locomotion of lame birds 1 h after treatment	PD	27
Flunixin meglumide	5.0	IM	Single injection	Mallard ducks	12-h activity but muscle necrosis at injection site	PD	28
	5.5	IM	24 for 7 days	Budgerigars	Severe renal lesions	TOX	29
	1.1	IV	Single injection	Chickens, ostrich, ducks, turkeys, pigeons	Chickens had long half-life but 10 min $t_{1/2}$ in ostrich	PK	25
	3	IM	Single injection	Chickens	Arthritis painful behaviors reduced 1 h after treatment	PD	24

Drug	Dose	Route	Interval	Species	Comments	Type	Reference
Ketoprofen	2.0	IV, IM, oral	Single injection	Quail	Low bioavailability IM, orally. Short IV $t_{1/2}$	PK	30
	12	IM	Single injection	Chickens	Arthritis painful behaviors reduced 1 h after treatment	PD	24
	2.5	IM	24 for 7 days	Budgerigars	Renal tubular necrosis	TOX	29
	5	IM	Single injection	Mallard ducks	12-h activity	PD	28
	2.0	Oral	12–24	Eiders	Mortality associated with male eiders	CS	31
	5.0	IM, IV					
Meloxicam	1	IM	12	Hispaniolan Amazon parrots	Improved weight bearing on arthritic limb	PD	32
	0.1	IM	24 for 7 days	Budgerigars	Renal glomerular congestion	TOX	29
	0.5	IV	Single injection	Chickens, ostrich, ducks, turkeys, pigeons	Variable distribution, slow clearance except ostrich	PK	25
	2	IM, oral	Single treatment	Cape Griffon vultures	Short $t_{1/2}$, less than 45 min	PK	33
Piroxicam	0.5–0.8	Oral	12	Whooping cranes	Used for acute myopathy and chronic arthritis	CS	J. Paul-Murphy, personal communication, July 1, 2010

Abbreviations: ASA, acetylsalicylic acid (aspirin); CS, care report or case series; IM, intramuscularly; IV, intravenously; PD, pharmacodynamic; PK, pharmacokinetic; TOX, toxicity; $t_{1/2}$, half-life.

contribute to postoperative pain. This noxious stimulus-induced sensitization can be prevented or preempted by administration of analgesic agents before tissue injury. This concept is being applied clinically with increasing frequency. Preemptive analgesia with opiates, NSAIDs, and/or local anesthetics can block sensory noxious stimuli from onward transmission to the CNS, thus reducing the overall potential for pain and inflammation, and potentially improving the patient's short-term and long-term recovery.

OPIOIDS

Opioids are used for moderate to severe pain, such as traumatic or surgical pain. Opioids reversibly bind to specific receptors in the central and peripheral nervous system. These drugs are categorized as either agonists, partial agonists, mixed agonist/antagonists, or antagonists based on their ability to induce an analgesic response once bound to a specific receptor. These drugs may be agonists at one receptor type and display antagonist or partial agonist effects at another receptor type. The agonist drugs have a linear dose-response curve that may be titrated to reach the desired effect, whereas the agonist/antagonist drugs may reach a ceiling effect after which increasing the dose does not seem to provide additional analgesia. During anesthesia, opioids are used to provide perioperative analgesia that may reduce the concentrations of volatile anesthetics (ie, gas anesthesia-sparing effects). The most common adverse effects reported with opioids are cardiac and/or respiratory depression. In many cases, these drugs may be reversed with antagonists, which will also terminate analgesia. The application and doses of several opioid formulations have been scientifically evaluated and clinically applied in birds (see **Table 1**).

Most opioid analgesics are used parenterally because of poor oral bioavailability associated with the first pass effect. Once absorbed, oral opioids first pass through the liver where they are metabolized, releasing a significantly lower amount of active drug into the general circulation. For example, the bioavailability of 5 mg/kg orally administered butorphanol in Hispaniolan Amazon parrots (*Amazona ventralis*) was less than 10% making this route ineffective (see **Table 1**).[12]

Opioids vary in their receptor specificity and efficacy in mammals, which results in a wide variety of clinical effects in different species. It is reasonable to presume that this opioid variability will also have a wide range of clinical effects in avian species. The distribution of opiate receptor types is well conserved across all mammalian species in the brainstem and spinal cord, but may vary markedly in the forebrain and midbrain. However, even with receptor distribution information in some species, it is still difficult to draw firm conclusions regarding the functional roles of different opioid receptor types because the physiologic and clinical effects of opioids may be influenced by pharmacologic variables such as the commercial preparation of opioid and the dose and route of administration, as well as by individual variables such as whether the animal has been stressed, injured, or anesthetized. There is an overall lack of published data concerning differences in opioid receptor distribution, density, and functionality in birds. In pigeons, the regional distribution of μ, κ, and δ receptors in the forebrain and midbrain were similar to mammals but the κ and δ receptors were more prominent in the pigeon forebrain and midbrain than μ receptors and 76% of opiate receptors in the forebrain were determined to be κ-type.[35] κ receptors have multiple physiologic functions in the bird and the analgesic function of these receptors still needs further investigation. It has been postulated that this difference in receptor distribution and density may partially explain why birds do not seem to respond to μ agonists in the same manner as mammals. However, in day-old chicks, marked dissimilarities to this distribution suggest either age- or species-related differences. It has been postulated that birds may not possess distinct μ and κ receptors or that the receptors may have similar functions. This may explain in part why the isoflurane-sparing effects of μ and κ agonists in chickens seemed to be similar to mammals.[36]

OPIOID FORMULATIONS

Morphine is a μ receptor agonist and has not been commonly used in avian medicine. Studies on domestic fowl have demonstrated confusing results on clinical doses. For example, morphine produced analgesia at high doses (200 mg/kg) in chicks in 1 early study using 1 testing strategy,[37] whereas later studies demonstrated analgesia with morphine in chicks at doses that approximate the analgesic dose range used in other species, however the results were sometimes conflicting.[2,38] Differing analgesic responses to morphine have also been detected between strains of chickens[39] including 1 study that showed analgesic effects in 1 strain at a given dose, whereas 2 other strains exhibited a hyperalgesic response with the same dose.[2] A study evaluating intraarticular injection of 1 to 3 mg morphine in a domestic fowl arthritis model found no significant antinociceptive effects but it is unclear whether pH differences in synovial fluid may have affected the activity of the drug.[20]

Fentanyl is a short-acting μ receptor agonist that has not been commonly used in avian medicine because historical investigations with morphine (the standard for μ opioids) administered to chickens were confusing and clinically inconclusive. Fentanyl 0.02 mg/kg intramuscularly (IM) did not affect the withdrawal thresholds to electrical or thermal stimuli of white cockatoos,[18] however, a tenfold increase in the dose (0.2 mg/kg subcutaneously [SC]) did produce an analgesic response, but many birds were hyperactive for the first 15 to 30 minutes after receiving the high dose.[18] Fentanyl had rapid absorption and elimination in parrots, with mean residence times of less than 2 hours (see **Table 1**).[18] Because of its short-acting properties, fentanyl delivered via constant-rate infusion (CRI) is an excellent choice as an analgesic adjunct to inhalant anesthesia in mammals and when used at low doses as a CRI, the authors have found fentanyl may also be effectively used in avian anesthetic protocols. Fentanyl administered as an intravenous (IV) CRI in red-tailed hawks (*Buteo jamaicensis*) to target plasma concentrations of 8 to 32 ng/mL reduced the minimum anesthetic dose (MAD) of isoflurane 31% to 55% in a dose-related manner, without statistically significant effects on heart rate, blood pressure, $Paco_2$, or Pao_2.[19] Fentanyl may also be combined with ketamine as a CRI thereby reducing the required doses of each.

Butorphanol is a mixed agonist/antagonist with low intrinsic activity at the μ receptor and strong agonist activity at the κ receptor. There is some evidence to suggest that butorphanol does not produce dose-related respiratory depression in contrast to μ receptor agonists. Adverse effects associated with butorphanol such as dysphoria have not been reported in birds. Preoperative butorphanol administration (2 mg/kg IM) did not show significant anesthetic (including time to intubation and extubation) or cardiopulmonary changes in Hispaniolan Amazon parrots anesthetized with sevoflurane, suggesting that it may be useful as part of a preemptive analgesic protocol (see **Table 1**).[17] Earlier isoflurane-sparing studies using 1 mg/kg IM butorphanol in cockatoos, African gray parrots (*Psittacus erithacus erithacus*), and blue-fronted Amazon parrots (*Amazona aestiva*) showed a significant reduction in the MAD for the cockatoos and African gray parrots, but not for the blue-fronted Amazon parrots, which indicates species variability at that dose of butorphanol (see **Table 1**).[14,15] In a study using withdrawal thresholds to electrical stimuli in conscious African gray parrots, butorphanol at 1 to 2 mg/kg showed a decreased withdrawal effect that was more significant at 2 mg/kg (see **Table 1**).[16] Butorphanol doses of 3 and 6 mg/kg IM had similar analgesic effects on Hispaniolan Amazon parrots (see **Table 1**).[16] Doses of 3 mg/kg demonstrated significant analgesia, but increasing the dose to 6 mg/kg did not increase the effect.[16] Based on these studies, doses of 1 to 4 mg/kg have been suggested in birds but empirical dosing frequencies ranging from 2 to 24 hours have been published. A recent study evaluating the PK of 0.5 mg/kg butorphanol in red-tailed hawks (*Buteo jamaicensis*) and great-horned owls (*Bubo virginianus*) found half-lives of 0.93 and 1.78 hours, respectively when given IV and 0.94 and 1.84 hours, respectively when given IM (see **Table 1**).[11] Likewise, low serum butorphanol concentrations were evident in Hispaniolan Amazon parrots 2 hours after single IM administration of a 5 mg/kg dose (see **Table 1**).[13] These data suggest that frequent dosing of butorphanol may be necessary in birds. This frequency of dosing is in some cases impractical because of lack of personnel to provide frequent dosing and the stress of frequent handling on the patient. A liposome-encapsulated, long-acting form of butorphanol tartrate was recently shown to be safe and effective in Hispaniolan parrots for up to 5 days following SC administration,[13] and was also shown to be an effective analgesic in Hispaniolan Amazon parrots and green-cheeked conures (*Pyrrhura molinae*) with induced arthritis.[26,34] The results from these studies are encouraging because a long-acting formulation of butorphanol would allow for both reduced frequency in butorphanol dosing and handling of avian patients for drug administration. Unfortunately, this formulation is not yet commercially available.

Buprenorphine is a slow-onset, long-acting opiate with a unique and complex pharmacologic profile. Buprenorphine is believed to act as a partial μ agonist but its κ receptor activities are less well defined. Several studies suggest that buprenorphine demonstrates κ receptor agonist effects but other evidence in mammals and pigeons suggests that it also displays some κ antagonistic activities. Buprenorphine has unusual receptor-binding characteristics that seem to be the result of slow drug dissociation from opioid receptors. Buprenorphine may exhibit a plateau or ceiling analgesic effect; increased doses may result in no additional analgesia, or may have detrimental effects. Few studies have been published evaluating the use of buprenorphine in birds. One study evaluating 0.05 to 1.0 mg buprenorphine administered intraarticularly in a domestic fowl arthritis model found no significant antinociceptive effects but it is unclear whether differences in the pH of synovial fluid may have affected the activity of the drug.[20] Buprenorphine at 0.1 mg/kg IM in African gray parrots did not have an analgesic effect when tested by PD analgesimetry, but PK analysis suggests this dose did not achieve plasma concentrations effective for humans (see **Table 1**).[16,21] Pigeons given 0.25 and 0.5 mg/kg IM buprenorphine had an increased latency period for withdrawal from a noxious electrical stimulus of 2 and 5 hours, respectively.[22] Further work is required to determine whether clinical efficacy may be obtained using different buprenorphine doses in other avian species.

Nalbuphine hydrochloride exerts its agonist activity principally at the κ receptor and is a partial antagonist at the μ receptor. It is used as an analgesic in the treatment of moderate to severe pain in humans and has a relatively lower incidence of respiratory depression that does not increase with additional dosing. Nalbuphine hydrochloride was rapidly cleared after both IM and IV dosing of 12.5 mg/kg to Hispaniolan Amazon parrots and had excellent bioavailability following IM administration, with little sedation and no adverse effects (see **Table 1**).[40] The same dose increased threshold values of thermal foot withdrawal in this species for up to 3 hours; higher doses (25 and 50 mg/kg IM) did not significantly increase the withdrawal threshold values above those of the 12.5 mg/kg dose.[23] Because of its low abuse potential, this opioid is currently not a Drug Enforcement Administration scheduled substance. Based on the receptor activity of this drug, and its potential for minor to few side effects, nalbuphine hydrochloride may show promise as an analgesic in pain management protocols in avian patients.

NSAIDs

NSAIDs are the most common class of analgesic drugs prescribed in small animal medicine. NSAIDs are used to relieve musculoskeletal and visceral pain, acute pain, and chronic pain such as osteoarthritis. The pharmacologic activity of NSAIDs has been reviewed in veterinary articles and textbooks and although most reviews do not consider avian applications, it is assumed that the chemistry and mechanism of action is similar when administered to birds.[41,42] A broad tissue distribution of cyclooxygenase (COX) has been demonstrated in chickens.[43] The relative expression of COX-1 and COX-2 enzymes varies between species and both enzymes are important in avian pain, but more information is needed to differentiate their physiologic effects in avian species.

The application and doses of several NSAID formulations continues to be scientifically evaluated as well as clinically applied in birds (see **Table 2**). As new NSAID formulations appear on the human and veterinary pharmaceutical market, the off-label use of these drugs in birds will be apparent. The intention of recently developed NSAIDs has been to spare COX-1 and emphasize COX-2 inhibition with the goal of providing analgesia and suppressing inflammation without inhibiting physiologically important prostaglandins. The common NSAIDs used in avian medicine at the time of this writing include meloxicam, carprofen, ketoprofen, celecoxib, and piroxicam, each with a distinct COX-1/COX-2 ratio and differing reports of effectiveness and toxicity in birds.

The selection of NSAID is determined by the ease of administration best suited to the situation; for example, giving an injectable formulation at the time of surgery, followed by oral formulation of the same or different NSAID postoperatively. There is little scientific support for a washout period when switching NSAIDs.[41] In cases of acute or chronic pain there may be a benefit to changing the NSAID and a washout period could put the bird at risk of having untreated pain. Only 1 NSAID should be used at a time, but in cases of chronic pain the response to therapy needs to be frequently reevaluated and the NSAID may need to be changed or augmented with other analgesics if response is poor or diminishing.

To evaluate the analgesic efficacy of an NSAID for avian species, several criteria need to be considered. The dose and frequency of NSAID administration depends on PD evaluations as well as PK data. Plasma levels are not sufficient information to predict the physiologic activity of the NSAID. Antiinflammatory and analgesic effects of NSAIDs continue longer than predicted by plasma half-lives. One explanation for the long duration of effect is the high protein binding, such as the protein in an inflamed site, which acts as a reservoir for the drug after it has been eliminated from the plasma.[44] This leads to persistence of the NSAID in inflamed sites longer than in the plasma. An alternate explanation is possible biotransformation of NSAIDs leading to active metabolites not being measured, however, metabolism of most NSAIDs in mammalian species occurs in the liver and the metabolites are generally inactive, and it assumed to be similar in avian species. Most NSAIDs are weak acids that are highly protein bound and most have a small volume of distribution. There are tremendous species differences in drug elimination among the NSAIDs.

The best example of avian species variability is the PK study of meloxicam, flunixin, and sodium salicylate administered intravenously to chickens, ostriches (*Struthio camelus*), mallard ducks (*Anas platyrhynchos*), turkeys (*Meleagris gallopavo*), and pigeons (*Columba livia*).[25] All 3 NSAIDs were rapidly eliminated in these species, however the volume of distribution was highly variable, which may reflect species differences in protein binding. Allometric analysis of the NSAID data in these 5 species concluded that despite renal filtration of the drugs, allometry is not useful for extrapolation of doses between avian species.[25] Although the distribution, half-life, and clearance have been characterized for some NSAIDs in a few species of birds, this information has not always been of use for predicting safe and effective dose regimens.

Presently accepted PD NSAID studies measure inhibitory concentrations of COX-1 and COX-2 concurrent with the PK of the drug to derive the clinically optimal and safe doses for animals, but these studies have not been done in any avian species. However, PD studies have been published describing the effects of ketoprofen and flunixin on thromboxane B2 (TBX) concentrations in mallard ducks.[28] Because NSAIDs block binding of arachidonic acid with COX enzyme, preventing conversion to TBX, plasma TBX is used to estimate the duration of NSAID action. In mallard ducks, flunixin (5 mg/kg) and ketoprofen (5 mg/kg) suppressed TBX levels for up to 12 hours, suggesting that their physiologic action may be that long.[28,45] A field study using ketoprofen in mallard ducks demonstrated analgesic effects but noted that the onset of analgesic effects may be longer than 30 minutes in some ducks.[45]

In vivo measurements use analgesimetry to evaluate the effect of an NSAID under physiologic and pathologic conditions and predict clinical outcome. Several analgesimetry models have been used to evaluate the PD of NSAIDs in chickens. Dose responses for carprofen, flunixin, ketoprofen, and sodium salicylate for treatment of inflammatory pain were determined in chickens using the articular pain model to measure the effect on specific behaviors.[24] Sodium salicylate was determined to be less effective than the other NSAIDs and large doses of carprofen were needed to return to nonarthritic behaviors; minimum effective doses determined in this study are listed in **Table 2**. A similar experimental arthritis model in parrots (*Amazona ventralis*) was used to evaluate NSAID treatment by measuring the return to normal weight bearing.[26,32] Carprofen (2 mg/kg IM every 12 hours) was less effective than butorphanol to improve weight bearing on the arthritic limb in parrots.[26] Alternatively, in a similar study, meloxicam (1 mg/kg IM every 12 hours) was effective at returning the parrots to normal weight bearing on the arthritic limb throughout the 36 hours of observation.[32]

ADVERSE EFFECTS OF NSAIDs

The most common adverse actions of NSAIDS in mammals include effects on the gastrointestinal system, renal system, and coagulation. NSAIDs have recently been implicated in humans and mammals with an increased risk of myocardial infarction and delays in bone healing,[46,47] but these effects have not been substantiated in birds. However, it is prudent to be aware that these adverse effects are often dose dependent and associated with chronic administration. The most common adverse effect of NSAIDs reported in avian species is the effect on renal tissue and function.

Prostaglandins in the kidney have an important role in regulating water and mineral balances and modulating intravascular tone. The kidney uses both COX-1 and COX-2 for prostaglandin synthesis and injury occurs when renal prostaglandin synthesis is inhibited. Originally it was hypothesized that the adverse renal effects of NSAIDs were linked primarily to COX-1 inhibition, however COX-2–selective NSAIDs may also have a significant risk of inducing adverse effects. COX-2 is constitutively expressed in the kidney in chickens, similar to all mammalian species studied and is highly regulated in response to alterations in intravascular volume.[43] COX-2 metabolites have been implicated in the maintenance of renal blood flow, mediation of renin release, and regulation of sodium excretion. Therefore, in conditions of relative intravascular volume depletion and/or renal hypoperfusion such as dehydration, hemorrhage, hemodynamic compromise, heart failure, and renal disease, interference with COX-2 activity can have significant deleterious effects on renal blood flow and glomerular filtration rate. In a study using northern bobwhite quail (Colinus virginianus), birds were treated for 7 days with a range of flunixin meglumine doses and even the lowest dose (0.1 mg/kg) caused glomerular lesions.[48] When budgerigars were treated with 5.5 mg/kg flunixin meglumine, 2.5 mg/kg ketoprofen, or 0.1 mg/kg meloxicam for either 3 or 7 days, plasma uric acid and protein levels did not change but a low frequency of glomerular congestion, degeneration, and dilation of tubules occurred.[29] Lesions were more severe in birds treated with flunixin meglumine for 3 or 7 days with increased mesangial matrix synthesis.[29]

The recent massive mortalities in 3 vulture species on the Asian subcontinent led to banning of the NSAID diclofenac (DF) on the Indian subcontinent. Common findings of diffuse visceral gout and proximal convoluted tubular damage indicated that the site of toxicity was the kidneys or the renal supportive vascular system.[49,50,51,52] The association of DF with vulture mortalities led to several investigations to establish the mechanism of toxicity for DF and other NSAIDs in several avian species. The effect of DF on inhibition of renal prostaglandins and subsequent closure of the renal portal valves was proposed to cause severe renal ischemia and nephrotoxicity.[51] But recent studies determined that vulture susceptibility to DF results from a combination of an increased reactive oxygen species (chemically reactive molecules containing oxygen such as oxygen ions and peroxide), interference with uric acid transport, and the duration of exposure.[50] Both DF and meloxicam were found to be toxic to renal tubular epithelial cells following 12 hours of cell culture exposure, caused by an increase in production of reactive oxygen species; in cultures incubated with either drug for only 2 hours, meloxicam showed no toxicity in contrast to DF.[50] DF also decreased the transport of uric acid, by interfering with the p-amino-hippuric acid channel. In addition, the half-life of DF in vultures (14 hours) is much longer than chickens (2 hours) thus exposing vultures to toxic effects of DF for prolonged time periods.[50]

NSAID FORMULATIONS

Ketoprofen is a potent nonselective COX-1 inhibitor that has been used extensively in small animal medicine. The excellent oral bioavailability of ketoprofen in mammals makes this drug attractive for oral dosing. However, ketoprofen is most commonly used parenterally in birds because of limited oral PK data and difficulty in accurately dosing the oral formulation in small species. PK studies evaluating a single dose of 2 mg/kg ketoprofen given orally, IM, and IV in Japanese quail (Coturnix japonica) showed very low oral (24%) and IM (54%) bioavailability of the drug, and the shortest half-life reported for this NSAID in any species.[30] Although it is possible that drug formulation could account for the low bioavailability of the drug in this study, additional studies are needed to determine whether drug formulations or physiologic differences between species could account for these differences. PD studies of 5 mg/kg IM ketoprofen in mallard ducks (Anas platyrhynchos) found an overall decrease in the inflammatory mediator TBX for approximately 12 hours after administration.[28] This suggests that the duration of the antiinflammatory effect in the mallards may parallel that of some mammals studied, therefore further studies in additional species are necessary to evaluate the duration of effect and bioavailability of this drug in birds. When ketoprofen (2 to 5 mg/kg IM) was administered to free-ranging spectacled eiders (*Somateria fischeri*) and king eiders (*Somateria spectabilis*), 4/10 male spectacled eiders and 5/6 male king eiders died within 1 to 4 days after surgery.[31] The histologic findings included severe renal tubular necrosis, acute rhabdomyolysis, and mild visceral gout. Strong consideration was given to the male behaviors during the mating season that may have predisposed these birds to dehydration and the adverse effects of COX inhibition.[31]

Carprofen can be administered parenterally or orally and is well absorbed through the gastrointestinal tract in mammals. The mechanism of action of carprofen has not been fully elucidated. It is a weak inhibitor of COX at therapeutic doses and yet exhibits good antiinflammatory activity. This weak inhibition of both COX isoforms may explain its wide margin of safety compared with other NSAIDs and it may achieve its therapeutic effects partially through other pathways.[53] Carprofen given SC significantly improved the speed and walking ability of lame chickens in a dose-dependent manner[27] An extremely high dose of carprofen of 30 mg/kg IM was needed for analgesia in chickens with experimental arthritis[24]; this dose is 6 to 10 times higher than standard mammal doses. An analgesia study in Hispaniolan Amazon parrots with experimental arthritis noted that 2 hours after carprofen administration, lameness was markedly improved but the analgesic effect was very short-term because 3 mg/kg IM of carprofen every 12 hours did not significantly improve the weight-bearing load of the arthritic limb for the 30-hour study period.[26] It was noted that 2 hours after carprofen administration, the lameness was markedly improved but the analgesic effect was very short-term.[26] Much work is needed to determine appropriate doses, dosing routes, and dosing frequency of carprofen in birds.

Meloxicam is a COX-2 selective oxicam NSAID. In recent years, meloxicam has become the most widely used antiinflammatory medication in exotic animal practice. A survey to determine NSAID toxicity in captive birds treated in zoos reported zero fatalities associated with meloxicam, which was administered to more than 700 birds from 60 species.[54] Ostriches given meloxicam IV exhibited the most rapid half-life (0.5 hours) compared with ducks, turkeys, pigeons, and chickens.[25] Meloxicam is currently available as an oral suspension and an injectable form. A dose-response analgesia study with Hispaniolan Amazon parrots with experimental arthritis determined that 1 mg/kg of meloxicam IM every 12 hours was necessary to achieve significant return to baseline weight bearing.[32] Oral administration of 1 mg/kg of meloxicam suspension to Hispaniolan Amazon parrots had lower bioavailability than when administered parenterally, and the highest mean concentration expected to provide analgesia was 6 hours after administration.[55] Japanese quail were treated with 2mg/kg of meloxicam IM for 14 days and the changes in complete blood count and serum chemistry parameters were minimal; the histologic changes in the kidney were unremarkable.[56] Clinical recommendations for treatment of parrots with high doses of meloxicam needs critical examination of its effect on renal parenchyma. Future studies to evaluate PD-PK of meloxicam administered by different routes in different avian species is necessary to determine appropriate analgesic doses and dosing schedules for meloxicam in avian patients.

Piroxicam is a nonselective NSAID used for its antiinflammatory properties as well as its value as a chemopreventative and antitumor agent. It has a much higher potency against COX-1 than COX-2. Piroxicam has good oral bioavailability and a long half-life in mammals but PD and PK studies have not been done in any avian species. Despite the high incidence of the negative side effects of piroxicam used in humans, there are no reports of its toxicity in birds. It has been used clinically for long-term treatment of chronic arthritis in cranes.[57]

REGIONAL ANESTHESIA AND ANALGESIA

In all vertebrates, including birds, local anesthetics block sodium channels in the nerve axon, interfering with the generation and conduction of action potentials along the nerve. When local anesthetics are used preemptively, the number and frequency of impulses are reduced, thereby reducing nociceptor sensitization, which has the beneficial effect of minimizing central sensitization. Regional infiltration using a local line or splash block is the most common method. The subcutaneous space in most avian species is very thin so a small-gauge needle is recommended to make several SC injections into the operative area. Lidocaine and bupivacaine have been used for brachial plexus blockade in a variety of avian species but a recent evaluation of bupivacaine (2 and 8 mg/kg) and lidocaine with epinephrine (15 mg/kg) found neither to effectively block nerve transmission in the brachial plexus of mallard ducks,[58] which was similar to the significant failure rate reported when studied in chickens.[59] Local anesthetics in the form of transdermal patches and creams, epidural infusions, spinal blocks, and intravenous blocks have not been reported.

Local anesthetics are absorbed by the vasculature in the region being blocked. Systemic uptake of the local anesthetics can be rapid in birds, and metabolism may be prolonged, increasing the potential for toxic reactions. The duration of action depends on the molecular properties and lipid solubility of the drug. Neither the time to effect nor duration of action has been determined in birds. Dosage recommendations are lower for birds than mammals because birds may be more sensitive to the effects of the drug. Chickens given intraarticular injections of high doses of bupivacaine (2.7 to 3.3 mg/kg) showed immediate signs of toxicity such as drowsiness and recumbency.[60] Other toxic effects reported in birds include fine tremors, ataxia, recumbency, seizures, stupor, cardiovascular effects, and death. Toxic effects can be acute if accidentally injected intravenously.

Lidocaine is available as a commercial preparation of 2% (20 mg/mL) and the formulation without epinephrine is recommended. Based on empirical use, the recommended dose is 2 to 3 mg/kg, although 15 mg/kg with epinephrine had no adverse effects when used for brachial plexus block in mallard ducks.[58] For small birds, the commercial preparation may need to be diluted 1:10 or more to achieve an effective volume for the block. It is unknown whether this dilution provides either the appropriate tissue drug levels for analgesia or the expected duration of analgesia.

Bupivacaine is the most clinically useful perioperative local anesthetic in mammals because it is a long-acting local anesthetic. The commercial preparations of bupivacaine available are 0.25%, 0.5%, and 0.75% solutions (2.5, 5, 7.5 mg/mL, respectively), and the lower concentration may not need dilution for birds. It has been used conservatively in birds because of concerns that toxic effects may take longer to resolve as a result of this drug's longer duration of effect. The recommended maximum dose of bupivacaine for mammals is 2 mg/kg, however results from a study in which mallard ducks (*Anas platyrhynchos*) were given bupivacaine (2 mg/kg SC) suggested that bupivacaine may be shorter acting in ducks than in mammals.[61] In this study, bupivacaine showed a faster absorption versus elimination rate, and sequestration and redistribution of bupivacaine was suggested by increases in plasma concentrations at 6 and 12 hr after administration making it possible for toxicity to be delayed. Higher doses of 8 mg/kg had no adverse effects when used for brachial plexus block in ducks.[58] Intraarticular bupivacaine (3 mg in 0.3 mL saline) was effective for treating arthritic pain in 1.5-kg chickens.[60] A 1:1 mixture of bupivacaine and dimethyl sulfoxide was applied to amputated chicken beaks immediately after amputation and feed intake was improved.[62]

OTHER ANALGESICS

Tramadol hydrochloride is an analgesic that has become popular recently despite minimal evidence as to its efficacy. It is active at opiate, alpha-adrenergic, and serotonergic receptors.[63] Tramadol is a weak μ agonist but the O-desmethyl metabolite (M1) is a much more potent agonist in mammals. Other metabolites including M2-M5 have also been described but their analgesic properties, if any, are not yet known. The conversion to the M1 metabolite is variable among species but it is known that it is produced in bald eagles, red-tailed hawks, (Souza MJ, personal communication, July 1, 2010) and Hispaniolan Amazon parrots.[64,65] It is available in oral and injectable formulations and currently the drug is not a controlled substance. In humans, less respiratory depression and constipation are seen with tramadol than with μ agonist opioids, but there are no data to date for other species. The oral (11 mg/kg) and IV (4 mg/kg) pharmacokinetics of single-dose tramadol have been evaluated in bald eagles[65] but analgesic plasma concentrations for tramadol and its M1 metabolite have not yet been established. Oral bioavailability of tramadol (mean ± SD = 97.94 ± 0.52%) was higher than that observed in humans and dogs, suggesting this as a useful route of administration in this species. Tramadol 11 mg/kg administered orally achieved concentrations in the human analgesic range for 10 hours in 5/6 bald eagles; M1 plasma concentrations reached the human range only in 2 eagles at much earlier time points.[65] The $t_{1/2}$ of tramadol in bald eagles after oral dosing was 2 times that reported in dogs, but half as long as in humans.[65] Until specific analgesic plasma concentrations are known, it is difficult to predict how these differences may affect appropriate dosing frequency after repeated doses. Mild transient bradycardia was observed immediately after IV administration in 3/6 birds, but was not considered clinically significant.[65] Although this analgesic holds great promise for use in birds, much work is still needed to evaluate appropriate dosing, efficacy, and safety of this drug in different species.

Gabapentin, a γ-aminobutyric acid analogue, has been used to treat neuropathic pain in humans for almost a decade. Its exact mechanism of action is unknown, but its therapeutic action on neuropathic pain is believed to involve voltage-gated N-type calcium ion channels. To date, there is only 1 published report and 2 proceedings articles on the clinical use of gabapentin as part of a multimodal therapeutic plan for suspected neuropathic pain in birds.[66,67,68] In all 3 reports, self-mutilation appeared to be relieved after the addition of gabapentin to the therapeutic regime.

BALANCED OR MULTIMODAL ANALGESIA

Combinations of drugs acting at different points in the nociceptive system provide a greater effect and potentially less toxicity than individual drugs given alone. For example, opioids generally act centrally to limit the input of nociceptive information into the CNS, whereas NSAIDS generally act peripherally to decrease inflammation thus limiting the nociceptive information that initially enters the CNS. Balanced analgesia with opiates, NSAIDS and/or local anesthetics administered before a painful procedure can block sensory noxious stimuli from onward transmission to the CNS, thus reducing the overall potential for pain and inflammation. These synergies have been demonstrated in laboratory animals and are now being used in the clinical environment. Balanced analgesia should be considered in virtually every avian patient as the use of multimodal therapy may maximize analgesic efficacy and minimize individual drug toxicity in these patients for which few analgesic data are available.

SUMMARY

Avian analgesia is now recognized as a critical component of avian medicine and surgery. The need to recognize pain and to provide pain relief is the first step, and many anecdotal therapeutic doses have been extrapolated from other companion animals. Several published research investigations, using several species of birds, have begun to provide avian analgesia therapeutic information for clinical application. The challenge is to continue pushing this research forward with appreciation that there are approximately 10,000 known species of birds, perhaps 200 species commonly kept as pets, and that each species has a range of behaviors as varied as their species-specific PKs and PDs for each analgesic drug.

REFERENCES

1. Sufka KJ, Hoganson DA, Hughes RA. Central monoaminergic changes induced by morphine in hypoalgesic and hyperalgesic strains of domestic fowl. Pharmacol Biochem Behav 1992;42:781–5.
2. Hughes RA. Strain-dependent morphine-induced analgesic and hyperalgesic effects on thermal nociception in domestic fowl (Gallus gallus). Behav Neurosci 1990;104:619–24.
3. Heatley JJ, Oliver JW, Hosgood G, et al. Serum corticosterone concentrations in response to restraint, anesthesia, and skin testing in Hispaniolan Amazon parrots (Amazona ventralis). J Avian Med Surg 2000;14:172–6.
4. Le Maho Y, Karmann H, Briot D, et al. Stress in birds due to routine handling and a technique to avoid it. Am J Physiol Regul Integr Comp Physiol 1992;263: 775–81.
5. Mathews KA. Pain assessment and general approach to management. Vet Clin North Am Small Anim Pract 2000;30:729–55.
6. Gentle MJ, Hill FL. Oral lesions in the chicken: behavioural responses following nociceptive stimulation. Physiol Behav 1987;40:781–3.
7. Gentle MJ, Hunter LN. Physiological and behavioural responses associated with feather removal in Gallus gallus var domesticus. Res Vet Sci 1991;50:95–101.
8. Graham DL. Pet birds: historical and modern perspectives on the keeper and the kept. J Am Vet Med Assoc 1998;212:1216–9.
9. Gentle MJ, Tilston VL. Reduction in peripheral inflammation by changes in attention. Physiol Behav 1999;66:289–92.
10. Lees P. Veterinary advances in PK/PD modelling. J Vet Pharmacol Ther 2004; 27:395.
11. Riggs SM, Hawkins MG, Craigmill AL, et al. Pharmacokinetics of butorphanol tartrate in red-tailed hawks (Buteo jamaicensis) and great horned owls (Bubo virginianus). Am J Vet Res 2008;69:596–603.
12. Sanchez-Migallon GD, Paul-Murphy J, Barker S, et al. Plasma concentrations of butorphanol in Hispaniolan Amazon parrots (Amazona ventralis) after intravenous and oral administration. Proc Assoc Avian Vet Conf 2008;23–4.
13. Sladky KK, Krugner-Higby L, Meek-Walker E, et al. Serum concentrations and analgesic effects of liposome-encapsulated and standard butorphanol tartrate in parrots. Am J Vet Res 2006;67:775–81.
14. Curro TG. Evaluation of the isoflurane-sparing effects of butorphanol and flunixin in psittaciformes. Proc Assoc Avian Vet Conf 1994;17–9.

15. Curro TG, Brunson DB, Paul-Murphy J. Determination of the ED50 of isoflurane and evaluation of the isoflurane-sparing effect of butorphanol in cockatoos (*Cacatua* spp). Vet Surg 1994;23:429–33.

16. Paul-Murphy J, Brunson DB, Miletic V. Analgesic effects of butorphanol and buprenorphine in conscious African grey parrots (*Psittacus erithacus erithacus* and *Psittacus erithacus timneh*). Am J Vet Res 1999;60:1218–21.

17. Klaphake E, Schumacher J, Greenacre C, et al. Comparative anesthetic and cardiopulmonary effects of pre- versus postoperative butorphanol administration in Hispaniolan Amazon parrots (*Amazona ventralis*) anesthetized with sevoflurane. J Avian Med Surg 2006;20:2–7.

18. Hoppes S, Flammer K, Hoersch K, et al. Disposition and analgesic effects of fentanyl in white cockatoos (*Cacatua alba*). J Avian Med Surg 2003;17:124–30.

19. Pavez JC, Pascoe PJ, DiMaio Kynch HK, et al. Effect of fentanyl target-controlled infusions on isoflurane MAD for red-tailed hawks (*Buteo jamaicensis*). Proc Assoc Avian Vet Conf 2010:29.

20. Gentle MJ, Hocking PM, Bernard R, et al. Evaluation of intraarticular opioid analgesia for the relief of articular pain in the domestic fowl. Pharmacol Biochem Behav 1999;63:339–43.

21. Paul-Murphy J, Hess J, Fialkowski JP. Pharmokinetic properties of a single intramuscular dose of buprenorphine in African grey parrots (*Psittacus erithacus erithacus*). J Avian Med Surg 2004;18:224–8.

22. Gaggermeier B, Henke J, Schatzmann U. Investigations on analgesia in domestic pigeons (*C. livia*, Gmel., 1789, var. dom.) using buprenorphine and butorphanol. Proc Eur Assoc Avian Vet Conf 2003;70–3.

23. Sanchez-Migallon GD, Keller D, KuKanich B, et al. Pharmacokinetics and antinociceptive effects of nalbuphine hydrochloride in Hispaniolan Amazon parrots (*Amazona ventralis*). Proc Assoc Avian Vet 2010;27–8.

24. Hocking PM, Robertson GW, Gentle MJ. Effects of non-steroidal anti-inflammatory drugs on pain-related behaviour in a model of articular pain in the domestic fowl. Res Vet Sci 2005;78:69–75.

25. Baert K, De Backer P. Comparative pharmacokinetics of three non-steroidal anti-inflammatory drugs in five bird species. Comp Biochem Physiol C Toxicol Pharmacol 2003;134:25–33.

26. Paul-Murphy JR, Sladky KK, Krugner-Higby LA, et al. Analgesic effects of carprofen and liposome-encapsulated butorphanol tartrate in Hispaniolan parrots (*Amazona ventralis*) with experimentally induced arthritis. Am J Vet Res 2009;70:1201–10.

27. McGeowen D, Danbury TC, Waterman-Pearson AE, et al. Effect of carprofen on lameness in broiler chickens. Vet Rec 1999;144:668–71.

28. Machin KL, Tellier LA, Lair S, et al. Pharmacodynamics of flunixin and ketoprofen in mallard ducks (*Anas platyrhynchos*). J Zoo Wildl Med 2001;32:222–9.

29. Pereira ME, Werther K. Evaluation of the renal effects of flunixin meglumine, ketoprofen and meloxicam in budgerigars (*Melopsittacus undulatus*). Vet Rec 2007;160:844–6.

30. Graham JE, Kollias-Baker C, Craigmill AL, et al. Pharmacokinetics of ketoprofen in Japanese quail (*Coturnix japonica*). J Vet Pharmacol Ther 2005;28:399–402.

31. Mulcahy DM, Tuomi P, Larsen RS. Differential mortality of male spectacled eiders (*Somateria fischeri*) and king eiders (*Somateria spectabilis*) subsequent to anesthesia with propofol, bupivacaine and ketoprofen. J Avian Med Surg 2003;17:117–23.

32. Cole GA, Paul-Murphy J, Krugner-Higby L, et al. Analgesic effects of intramuscular administration of meloxicam in Hispaniolan parrots (*Amazona ventralis*) with experimentally induced arthritis. Am J Vet Res 2009;70:1471–6.
33. Naidoo V, Wolter K, Cromarty AD, et al. The pharmacokinetics of meloxicam in vultures. J Vet Pharmacol Ther 2008;31:128–34.
34. Paul-Murphy JR, Krugner-Higby LA, Tourdot RL, et al. Evaluation of liposome-encapsulated butorphanol tartrate for alleviation of experimentally induced arthritic pain in green-cheeked conures (*Pyrrhura molinae*). Am J Vet Res 2009; 70:1211–9.
35. Mansour A, Khachaturian H, Lewis ME, et al. Anatomy of CNS opioid receptors. Trends Neurosci 1988;11:308–14.
36. Concannon KT, Dodam JR, Hellyer PW. Influence of a mu- and kappa-opioid agonist on isoflurane minimal anesthetic concentration in chickens. Am J Vet Res 1995;56:806–11.
37. Schneider C. Effects of morphine-like drugs in chicks. Nature 1961;191:607–8.
38. Hughes RA. Codeine analgesia and morphine hyperalgesia effects on thermal nociception in domestic fowl. Pharmacol Biochem Behav 1990;35:567–70.
39. Fan S, Shutt AJ, Vogt M. The importance of 5-hydroxytryptamine turnover for the analgesic effect of morphine in the chicken. Neuroscience 1981;6:2223–7.
40. Keller D, Sanchez-Migallon GD, Klauer J, et al. Pharmacokinetics of nalbuphine HCl in Hispaniolan Amazon parrots (*Amazona ventralis*). Proc Am Assoc Zoo Vet Conf 2009;106.
41. Papich MG. An update on nonsteroidal anti-inflammatory drugs (NSAIDs) in small animals. Vet Clin North Am Small Anim Pract 2008;38:1243–66, vi.
42. Bergh MS, Budsberg SC. The coxib NSAIDs: potential clinical and pharmacologic importance in veterinary medicine. J Vet Intern Med 2005;19:633–43.
43. Mathonnet M, Lalloue F, Danty E, et al. Cyclo-oxygenase 2 tissue distribution and developmental pattern of expression in the chicken. Clin Exp Pharmacol Physiol 2001;28:425–32.
44. Lees P, Landoni MF, Giraudel J, et al. Pharmacodynamics and pharmacokinetics of nonsteroidal anti-inflammatory drugs in species of veterinary interest. J Vet Pharmacol Ther 2004;27:479–90.
45. Machin KL, Livingston A. Assessment of the analgesic effects of ketoprofen in ducks anesthetized with isoflurane. Am J Vet Res 2002;63:821–6.
46. Gerstenfeld LC, Thiede M, Seibert K, et al. Differential inhibition of fracture healing by non-selective and cyclooxygenase-2 selective non-steroidal anti-inflammatory drugs. J Orthop Res 2003;21:670–5.
47. Dajani EZ, Islam K. Cardiovascular and gastrointestinal toxicity of selective cyclo-oxygenase-2 inhibitors in man. J Physiol Pharmacol 2008;59(Suppl 2): 117–33.
48. Klein PN, Charmatz K, Langenberg J. The effect of flunixin meglumine (banamine) on the renal function of northern bobwhite quail (*Colinus virginianus*): an avian model. Proc Am Assoc Zoo Vet 1994:128–31.
49. Oaks JL, Gilbert M, Virani MZ, et al. Diclofenac residues as the cause of vulture population decline in Pakistan. Nature 2004;427:630–3.
50. Naidoo V, Swan GE. Diclofenac toxicity in Gyps vulture is associated with decreased uric acid excretion and not renal portal vasoconstriction. Comp Biochem Physiol C Toxicol Pharmacol 2008;149:269–74.
51. Meteyer CU, Rideout BA, Gilbert M, et al. Pathology and proposed pathophysiology of diclofenac poisoning in free-living and experimentally exposed oriental white-backed vultures (*Gyps bengalensis*). J Wildl Dis 2005;41:707–16.

52. Swan GE, Cuthbert R, Quevedo M, et al. Toxicity of diclofenac to Gyps vultures. Biol Lett 2006;2:279–82.
53. Lees P, Landoni MF. Pharmacodynamics and enantioselective pharmacokinetics of racemic carprofen in the horse. J Vet Pharmacol Ther 2002;25:433–48.
54. Cuthbert R, Parry-Jones J, Green RE, et al. NSAIDs and scavenging birds: potential impacts beyond Asia's critically endangered vultures. Biol Lett 2007;3:90–3.
55. Molter C, Court M, Cole GA, et al. Pharmacokinetics of parenteral and oral meloxicam in Hispaniolan parrots (Amazona ventralis). Proc Assoc Avian Vet Conf 2009;317.
56. Sinclair K, Paul-Murphy J, Church M, et al. Renal physiologic and histopathologic effects of meloxicam in Japanese quail (Coturnix japonica). Proc Assoc Avian Vet Conf 2010;287.
57. Hanley CS, Thomas NJ, Paul-Murphy J, et al. Exertional myopathy in whooping cranes (Grus americana) with prognostic guidelines. J Zoo Wildl Med 2005;36: 489–97.
58. Brenner DJ, Larsen RS, Dickinson PJ, et al. Development of an avian brachial plexus nerve block technique for perioperative analgesia in mallard ducks (Anas platyrhynchos). J Avian Med Surg 2010;24:24–34.
59. Figueiredo JP, Cruz ML, Mendes GM, et al. Assessment of brachial plexus blockade in chickens by an axillary approach. Vet Anaesth Analg 2008;35:511–8.
60. Hocking PM, Gentle MJ, Bernard R, et al. Evaluation of a protocol for determining the effectiveness of pretreatment with local analgesics for reducing experimentally induced articular pain in domestic fowl. Res Vet Sci 1997;63:263–7.
61. Machin KL, Livingston A. Plasma bupivacaine levels in mallard ducks (Anas platyrhynchos) following a single subcutaneous dose. Proc Am Assoc Zoo Vet Conf 2001;159–63.
62. Glatz PC, Murphy LB, Preston AP. Analgesic therapy of beak-trimmed chickens. Aust Vet J 1992;69:18.
63. Scott LJ, Perry CM. Tramadol: a review of its use in perioperative pain. Drugs 2000;60:139–76.
64. Souza MJ, Sanchez-Migallon GD, Paul-Murphy J, et al. Tramadol in Hispaniolan Amazon parrots (Amazona ventralis). Proc Assoc Avian Vet Conf 2010;293–4.
65. Souza MJ, Martin-Jimenez T, Jones MP, et al. Pharmacokinetics of intravenous and oral tramadol in the bald eagle (Haliaeetus leucocephalus). J Avian Med Surg 2009;23:247–52.
66. Shaver SL, Robinson NG, Wright BD, et al. A multimodal approach to management of suspected neuropathic pain in a prairie falcon (Falco mexicanus). J Avian Med Surg 2009;23:209–13.
67. Siperstein LJ. Use of Neurontin (gabapentin) to treat leg twitching/foot mutilation in a Senegal parrot. Proc Assoc Avian Vet Conf 2007;335.
68. Doneley B. The use of gabapentin to treat presumed neuralgia in a little corella (Cacatua sanguinea). Proc Australian Assoc Avian Vet Conf 2007;169–72.

Rodent Analgesia

Amy L. Miller, PhD[a,b], Claire A. Richardson, BVM&S, MRCVS[a,b],*

KEYWORDS

- Rodent • Analgesia • Mice • Rats • Guinea pigs • Chinchillas

Rodents of all species are frequently kept as companion animals, with increasing client expectations for the care of their animals. Fortunately, specialist veterinary interest and information is now available for treatment of rodents. In the field of rodent analgesia particularly, much can be learned from the methods developed for preventing and alleviating pain in animals undergoing research studies in laboratories throughout the world. This article reviews advances in pain detection techniques in rodents and makes recommendations on analgesic agents that are available for the alleviation of pain.

RECOGNIZING PAIN

To effectively alleviate pain in animals we must first be able to recognize it. Recognition of pain and its intensity allows assessment of employed analgesic regimens to ensure that the treatments are both effective and appropriate. As animals cannot report the intensity of their pain, alternative methods of pain assessment must be used. Although this remains a challenge in veterinary practice, an awareness of ongoing research in pain assessment in animals can help us to detect and alleviate pain in pet rodents.

Objective Indicators of Pain in Animals

Objective methods of assessing pain are essential to ensure appropriate pain relief is provided. These methods often include monitoring food and water consumption along with any changes in body weight. Although pain is often associated with weight loss due to anorexia and a decrease in fluid consumption, these measures must be obtained retrospectively and therefore cannot be used to improve the analgesic therapy for that particular animal. However, information can be obtained with respect to specific procedures in that species, which can aid in the treatment of future animals.

Heart rate and respiratory rate have been used as an indirect measure of pain, with increases in both thought to accompany pain states[1]; however such measures should

The authors have nothing to disclose.

[a] Institute of Neuroscience, Medical School, Newcastle University, Framlington Place, Newcastle upon Tyne, Tyne and Wear, NE2 4HH, UK

[b] Comparative Biology Centre, Medical School, Newcastle University, Framlington Place, Newcastle upon Tyne, Tyne and Wear, NE2 4HH, UK

* Corresponding author. Institute of Neuroscience, Medical School, Newcastle University, Framlington Place, Newcastle upon Tyne, Tyne and Wear, NE2 4HH, UK.

E-mail address: claire.richardson@ncl.ac.uk

doi:10.1016/j.cvex.2010.09.004
1094-9194/11/$ – see front matter © 2011 Elsevier Inc. All rights reserved.

vetexotic.theclinics.com

be interpreted with caution, as many other factors can influence these parameters. Any stress or excitement, even handing the animal, will increase both heart rate and respiratory rate.[2] Obtaining heart rate and respiratory rates is not only difficult in awake rodents; resting heart rates may be too high to assess by auscultation or palpation of the pulse (eg, >300–400 beats/min).

Clinical Impression of the Animal

In practice the decision to administer an analgesic is often based largely on the veterinarian's clinical impression of an animal. Although not specific, an observation of a change in appearance or behavior in an animal following surgery or in painful conditions often indicates the presence of pain. As the response to pain varies considerably both between species and between individual animals, it is important that pain assessment is performed by clinicians with a comprehensive knowledge of the normal behavior and appearance of the species and animal concerned. These individuals will be the most likely to detect deviations from normal appearance and behavior in the animal. Monitoring at regular intervals is also imperative to ensure continued effective management of pain, particularly in the immediate hours following surgery or injury. Because different assessors may evaluate differently whether an animal is in pain, successive observations by a single observer are likely to provide the best insight into the improvement of an animal over time.

Although the use of pain-scoring scales has not been validated in rodents, it is likely that the use of these systems is preferable to simple observation. Descriptive, numerical, and visual analog (VAS) scales could all be used, but current opinion suggests that VAS may be the most useful in both animals and human infants.[3]

The presence of an observer may also affect the behavior of the animal; for example, many rabbits and guinea pigs often remain immobile.[4] This behavior may be a particular problem when the animal is observed by an unfamiliar person in an unfamiliar environment. It may therefore be beneficial to initially observe such animals from behind a viewing panel or via a video link. A simple web-cam provides an inexpensive means of making these observations.

In summary, while not specific, changes in general appearance and behavior in situations when pain is likely to occur are often indicative of pain. The administration of an analgesic and subsequent prevention or reversal of these behavioral changes can aid in the confirmation of pain. Unfortunately this can be challenging, because analgesics have been shown to influence the behavior of normal animals; for example, administration of buprenorphine leads to increased activity in normal mice.[5] These nonspecific analgesic effects on behavior must be taken into account when assessing the effectiveness of an analgesic.

Behavior-Based Pain-Scoring Systems

Behavior-based pain-scoring systems have been used successfully to study pain in many species. Behaviors such as lip licking, cage circling, and "flank gazing" have been observed in dogs after ovariohysterectomy accompanied by an increase in plasma cortisol, and have been attributed to the presence of pain.[6,7] Similarly, in combination with physiologic measures such as changes in plasma cortisol, specific behavioral responses have been observed in lambs and calves following castration and tail docking.[8,9] Behavior-based pain-scoring systems are now available for many species.[10]

Assessment of Rodents

Rodents do exhibit some signs of pain that are similar to those shown by other animals, including reflex withdrawal responses and vocalizations,[11] yet their specific responses to pain vary. It has been suggested that prey animals such as rats and mice deliberately attempt to disguise behavioral signs of pain to prevent unwanted attention from predators.[12,13] It may also be important for rodents not to show signs of weakness to cage mates to maintain their social status.[14] However, signs of pain in many species are subtle, with the exception of guarding behavior, such as observed with an injured limb. Once key behaviors that are likely to be associated with pain have been identified, it becomes reasonably easy to make an assessment of the intensity of pain being experienced by the animal. However, as mentioned earlier, familiarity with normal behavior is particularly important.

Clinical signs that may indicate pain in rodents are summarized in **Table 1**. In brief, these can include a decrease in general locomotion and a decrease in food and water consumption, with rapid weight loss an important concern. When group-housed, animals in pain may separate themselves from the rest of the group and, depending on cage layout, may remain in a corner or underneath the food hopper. The general appearance of the animal may also change, with it adopting a hunched posture and developing an unkempt coat (both due to piloerection and reduced grooming). When approached, rodents in pain may become unusually aggressive in an attempt to guard the painful area. Abnormal postures may also be more apparent during locomotion because alterations in posture during walking may be used to protect an injured area, for example, back arching[12] in rats and a raised tail position in mice.[15]

Assessment of Rats

In rats, porphyrin staining around the eyes is a nonspecific sign of stress that may indicate a painful state. The presence of porphyrin staining indicates that further pain assessment and a general clinical evaluation should be performed and that the animal should be carefully monitored.

Table 1
Clinical signs that may indicate pain in rodents

Clinical Sign	Description
Abnormal appearance	Lack of grooming Piloerection Hunched posture Porphyrin staining (rats)
Changes to normal behavior	Decrease in normal exploratory behaviors including walking, sniffing, and rearing Increase in other behaviors such as sleeping and time spent stationary Decrease in food and water consumption
Guarding	Alteration in body position or posture to prevent contact with a painful body part
Self mutilation	Excessive grooming, licking, biting, or scratching of the painful area
Vocalization	Particularly when the animal is handled or painful area is palpated Decrease in vocalizations may occur in guinea pigs
Specific behavioral changes	Twitching Abdominal contractions Back arching Belly pressing Walking with tail in a raised position (mice)

Successful behavior-based pain-scoring schemes for use in rats undergoing abdominal surgery have been developed.[12,16] Back arching, twitching, and abdominal contractions have been identified as behaviors that are infrequently observed before surgery, yet the frequency of these behaviors increases following abdominal surgery. Administration of a nonsteroidal anti-inflammatory drug (NSAID) such as carprofen or meloxicam, or an opioid such as buprenorphine decreases the occurrence of these behaviors postsurgically.[16,17]

Assessment of Mice

Following surgical procedures, mice are often fairly active within as little as 1 hour following recovery from anesthesia.[18] This observation has led to the assumption that pain relief may not be necessary, as they appear to behave in a normal manner almost immediately.[19] On closer observation, however, significant changes in behavior can be identified such as twitching, flinching, and writhing along, with a decrease in general exploratory behavior such as walking, rearing, and sniffing.[15,18,20,21]

A new potentially useful method of pain assessment in mice is through analysis of facial expressions. Facial expressions are often used successfully in human infants to assess pain. Recently, the use of facial expressions has been assessed in mice during periods when pain has been induced in laboratory studies.[22] Orbital tightening, nose bulges, cheek bulges, and changes in ear and whisker position have been linked to the presence of pain, and may be useful to indicate when further monitoring of an individual mouse is necessary. It is possible that similar changes may occur in other species.

Assessment of Guinea Pigs and Chinchillas

Limited work has been performed to date on pain assessment in guinea pigs and chinchillas. When handled, normal guinea pigs tend to squeal; however, those assumed to be experiencing pain tend to remain silent. Guinea pigs experiencing acute pain may also show changes in facial expression or aggression toward cage mates. As in other species, chronic pain may result in decreased responsiveness and anorexia.[23]

UNIQUE PHYSIOLOGY

As previously discussed, anorexia frequently occurs in painful conditions; this is particularly a problem in herbivorous rodents such as guinea pigs and chinchillas, which are prone to ileus following periods of anorexia.[24] Dehydration and hypoglycemia may occur in all rodents, so these animals should all be encouraged to eat. For mice and rats, provision of soaked diet on the floor of the cage may be beneficial, and all animals should be presented with a familiar favorite food. Guinea pigs and chinchillas should have good-quality hay readily available, and prokinetics may be administered. If these measures are not sufficiently effective, then syringe feeding may be required.

THERAPEUTICS

Analgesic dose rates based on body weight in rodents tend to be relatively high compared with other mammals, largely because of their small body size and fast metabolic rate. Dose rates of opioid agents given via the oral route are particularly high, due to the considerable first-pass metabolism by the liver (this topic is reviewed for mammalian species elsewhere in this issue).[25]

Systemic Analgesics

The 2 traditional classes of systemic analgesic agents used in rodents are opioids and NSAIDs.

Opioids

In brief, opioid analgesics include: (1) full agonists such as morphine, oxymorphone, hydromorphone, fentanyl, and alfentanil; (2) partial agonists such as buprenorphine; and (3) agonist-antagonists such as butorphanol. Morphine has long been considered to provide the gold standard in pain relief; however, there is sometimes reluctance to use it and the other opioid analgesics because of concerns about potential adverse effects. Although potential adverse effects of opioids such as respiratory depression, nausea,[26] gastrointestinal stasis,[27] and sedation should always be considered, they are often overestimated, and withholding analgesics for fear of adverse effects is not appropriate if animals are carefully monitored. It must be noted that buprenorphine, in common with other opioids, can be associated with pica (the ingestion of inedible substances such as bedding), particularly in rats.[28] If pica is observed, bedding may need to be temporarily removed and animals can be housed on other material to prevent gastric obstruction.

Nonsteroidal anti-inflammatory drugs

NSAIDs act by inhibiting cyclooxygenase (COX) enzymes that are involved in the production of the prostaglandins. Prostaglandins are produced in the first step of the synthesis of prostanoids, which act as mediators in the inflammatory pathway. NSAID activity largely targets the 2 isoforms COX-1 and COX-2.

The NSAID agents most frequently used in rodents include carprofen, meloxicam, and ketoprofen. NSAIDs traditionally have been recommended to alleviate mild pain; however, as the potency and COX selectivity of the newer agents has improved, they can now be used to alleviate more painful conditions. Unlike opioids, NSAIDs are not controlled drugs and may also provide a longer duration of action than many of the opioid agents.

Adverse effects from NSAID administration may target gastrointestinal and renal tissues, therefore NSAID administration is contraindicated in certain conditions such as chronic renal disease. In rodents the most frequently used NSAIDs such as carprofen, ketoprofen, and meloxicam appear to have a wide safety margin.[29–31] Adverse effects are most likely to occur following prolonged NSAID administration, which may be necessary as part of the management of chronic conditions such as arthritis and dental disease. Routine oral administration of low-dose meloxicam for prolonged periods appears to be well tolerated if animals are carefully monitored throughout the course of treatment.

Published analgesic dose rates for rodents tend to be based on either laboratory studies or anecdotal reports, but more reliable data based on postoperative pain assessment is beginning to emerge. Dose rates are summarized in **Table 2**, together with an indication of the quality of evidence supporting the recommendation. There is considerable variation between rodent strains and between individual animals, therefore patients should be carefully assessed (using the criteria outlined in the previous section) before and after analgesic administration.

To facilitate analgesic administration, some analgesic agents (eg, meloxicam) are available as palatable syrups that may be readily accepted by rodents using a small syringe. Analgesics may also be administered in food (eg, buprenorphine jelly)[25] or in drinking water (eg, acetaminophen [paracetamol]). Disadvantages of administration of analgesics via food or drinking water include inadequate dosing when pain results in anorexia and a reduction of drinking. Inadequate dosing will also occur if analgesics are unpalatable. Degradation by hydrolysis over time may also occur with analgesics in drinking water.[32] In addition, most rodents show marked diurnal patterns of water consumption, which would result in prolonged periods during which analgesics would

Table 2
Rodent analgesic dose rates

Drug	Dose (mg/kg)	Route	Interval (hours)	References
A. Rat				
Opioids				
Buprenorphine	0.01–0.05[a]	SC	8–12	17
	0.1–0.25	PO	8–12	10
Butorphanol	1.0–2.0	SC	4	10,19,44
Morphine	2.5	SC	4	10,19,44
Oxymorphone	0.2–0.5	SC		10,44,45
Tramadol	5	SC		10
NSAIDs				
Acetaminophen (paracetamol)	200	PO		10
Carprofen	5.0[a]	SC	12–24	12
	1.0–5.0	PO	12–24	46
Flunixin	2.5	SC		10,44,45
Ketoprofen	5.0[a]	SC		12
Meloxicam	1.0[a]	SC PO	12–24	16
B. Mice				
Opioids				
Buprenorphine	0.05–0.1	SC	12	10,19,44–46
Butorphanol	1.0–2.0	SC	4	10,19,44–46
Morphine	2.5	SC	2–4	10
Oxymorphone	0.2–0.5	SC		10,44
Tramadol	5.0	SC		10
NSAIDs				
Acetaminophen (paracetamol)	200	PO		10
Carprofen	5.0	SC	12–24	10,44,45

	Dose	Route	Interval (h)	References
Flunixin	2.5	SC		10,44,45
Ketoprofen	5	SC		10
Meloxicam	5[a]	SC, PO	24	10,21
C. Guinea Pigs				
Opioids				
Buprenorphine	0.05	SC	8–12	10,44–46
Butorphanol	1.0–2.0	SC	4	10,44
Morphine	2.0–5.0	SC, IM	4	10,46
Oxymorphone	0.2–0.5	SC		10,44
NSAIDs				
Carprofen	4.0	SC	12–24	10,44
Flunixin	2.5	SC		10,44
Ketoprofen	1.0	SC	12–24	45
Meloxicam	0.1–0.3	SC, PO	24	10,46
D. Chinchillas				
Opioids				
Buprenorphine	0.01–0.05	SC	6–12	44,46
Butorphanol	0.2–2.0	SC	2–4	44–46
NSAIDs				
Carprofen	4.0	SC	24	45
Ketoprofen	1.0	SC	12–24	45,46
Meloxicam	0.1–0.3	SC, PO	24	46

"_" indicates that information is insufficient to make a firm recommendation of an appropriate dose.

Abbreviations: IM, intramuscular; PO, per os (orally); SC, subcutaneous.

[a] Indicates a dose rate based on objective assessment of postoperative pain.

not be consumed. It is therefore recommended that the use of medicated water is always accompanied by other methods of treatment to ensure that analgesia is adequate. When analgesics are administered by injection, the subcutaneous route is generally preferable, as this route is well tolerated by the animal and particularly easy for the operator. The intramuscular route should be avoided or used with caution because of the small muscle mass and, therefore, potential for damage in rodents.

Preventive (or Preemptive) Analgesia

Preventive (formerly termed preemptive) analgesia should be used whenever possible when postsurgical pain is anticipated. Advantages of preventive analgesia include both the reduction of noxious stimuli reaching the central nervous system during surgery and the reduction of peripheral inflammation.[10] The administration of some opioids such as buprenorphine before surgery will have an anesthetic-sparing effect, reducing the dose of anesthetic required during surgery.[33] This effect can easily be incorporated into the anesthetic plan when using inhalant anesthetics; for example, buprenorphine 30 minutes preoperatively allows a reduction of isoflurane maintenance concentrations by about 0.25% to 0.5%.[34] When using injectable anesthetic agents, the effects can be less predictable, so opioid administration before the use of these agents should be performed with caution.[35] Preoperative NSAIDs are usually well tolerated in the well-hydrated patient; however, the potential adverse effects previously discussed may be a concern. Although preventive analgesia is preferable with respect to the efficacy of the agents, drug administration can be challenging and stressful to rodents because of their small size. Analgesics are therefore often combined with anesthetic agents and given as a single injection.[10]

Multimodal Analgesia

Multimodal analgesia refers to the use of different classes of analgesic agents and different sites of administration used to provide more effective analgesia. As nociception involves numerous different mechanisms, the use of multiple analgesics that act in different ways is likely to enhance pain relief. Adverse effects can also be minimized through use of lower doses of each individual drug. An example of a multimodal analgesic regimen for rodents undergoing surgery is to administer buprenorphine preoperatively, infiltrate the surgical field with lidocaine intraoperatively, and administer meloxicam postoperatively.

Local Anesthetics

Local anesthetic agents may be administered: (1) topically (eg, as a cream to facilitate venipuncture),[36] (2) locally by infiltration of the surgical site, (3) in peripheral nerve blocks, or (4) in epidural or spinal anesthesia. Lidocaine and bupivacaine are the most frequently used agents, with bupivacaine having a higher potency and longer duration of action but greater toxicity.

The toxicity of local anesthetics is very similar in large and small mammals; however, the small size of many rodent species makes inadvertent overdose a much more significant hazard. To minimize this risk when using local anesthetics, it is advisable to draw up the maximum safe dose before administration—approximately 10 mg/kg for lidocaine and 2 mg/kg for bupivacaine.[10] Further information on local anesthesia and techniques for performing intratesticular blocks and 5 types of dental blocks are described by Lichtenberger and Ko.[37]

Epidural Analgesia

Opioids may be combined with local anesthetics or administered as single agents via the epidural route. Studies performed in humans suggest that the analgesia produced via the epidural route is likely to be very effective,[38] and although technically challenging this technique is possible in rodents.[39]

Constant-Rate Infusions

Analgesics may be administered to effect when given via constant-rate infusion rather than as a bolus. This route has the advantage of allowing the clinician to minimize the total amount of analgesic used and therefore reduce potential side effects.[37] Constant-rate infusions also avoid "peaks and valleys" in drug concentration and are a valuable component of multimodal analgesia in many veterinary species.[40] Agents that may be used include opioids, ketamine, and α2-adrenoreceptor agonists. Although the use of constant-rate infusions is not frequently reported in companion rodents, this technique is used in the research environment.[41]

Relevance of Studies in Laboratory Animals

Much of what was originally published on the veterinary care of rodents has been based on rodents kept in laboratories. Analgesics available for clinical use have all undergone preclinical testing in laboratory rodents, therefore considerable information about the safety and efficacy of these agents is available and can be referred to when treating pet rodents. This information is valuable in the treatment of companion animal rodent cases. Three factors should remain in consideration when applying findings from laboratory studies: (1) licensing regulations, (2) translation of laboratory studies based on analgesiometry to clinical pain, and (3) differences between pet and laboratory rodent populations.

Licensing
The number of agents approved for domestic rodents is limited despite the copious amount of information on the safety of analgesic agents from laboratory animals. In the United States there are no drugs approved for use in domestic rodents, and only a limited number of licensed products are available within the United Kingdom.[42] Licensing regulations for "off-label use," permitted in the United States by the Animal Medicinal Drug Use Clarification Act of 1994, should be assessed and discussed with the pet owner prior to administration.

Translation of laboratory studies based on analgesiometric studies to clinical pain
Preclinical testing of analgesic agents on laboratory rodents typically involves assessment of acute pain responses through a variety of analgesiometric tests. Analgesiometric tests typically examine the response to a briefly painful mechanical, thermal, or electrical stimulus, and have been reviewed by Mogil.[43] Although the use of these tests often provides a safe and likely effective dose range for analgesic agents, the dose rates of analgesics that alter responses in analgesiometric tests are not always the most appropriate for treating clinical pain.[10]

Differences between pet and laboratory rodent populations
Laboratory studies are usually performed in young, healthy, adult strains of mice and rats. Dose rate may often need to be adjusted for companion animal rodents, which are often geriatric and may have concurrent diseases. Limited information is available about rodent species such as chinchillas and guinea pigs, which are less frequently used in laboratories.

ADDITIONAL CONCERNS

When considering postoperative pain, environmental factors and supportive care should always be considered. To minimize stress, rodents should be housed away from the sight and smells of their natural predators, including dogs, cats, ferrets, and raptors. Socially housed animals should also ideally be housed with their cage mates. As previously discussed, the use of a viewing panel or video link should be considered for postoperative assessment when monitored by unfamiliar individuals.

ACKNOWLEDGMENTS

The authors would like to thank Professor Paul Flecknell for his helpful comments on this article.

REFERENCES

1. Colpaert FC, Tarayre JP, Alliaga M, et al. Opiate self-administration as a measure of chronic nociceptive pain in arthritic rats. Pain 2001;91:33–45.
2. Livingston A, Chambers P. The physiology of pain. In: Flecknell P, Waterman-Pearson A, editors. Pain management in animals. London: WB Saunders; 2000. p. 9–20.
3. Price DD, Bush FM, Long S, et al. A comparison of pain measurement characteristics of mechanical visual analogue and simple numerical rating scales. Pain 1994;56:217–26.
4. Dobromylskyj P, Flecknell P, Lascelles BD, et al. Pain assessment. In: Flecknell P, Waterman-Pearson A, editors. Pain management in animals. London: WB Saunders; 2000. p. 53–80.
5. Cowan A, Doxey JC, Harry EJ. The animal pharmacology of buprenorphine, an oripavine analgesic agent. Br J Pharmacol 1977;60:547–54.
6. Fox SM, Mellor DJ, Stafford KJ, et al. The effects of ovariohysterectomy plus different combinations of halothane anaesthesia and butorphanol analgesia on behaviour in the bitch. Res Vet Sci 2000;68:265–74.
7. Hardie EM, Hansen BD, Carroll GS, et al. Behaviour after ovariohysterectomy in the dog: what's normal? Appl Anim Behav Sci 1997;51:111–28.
8. Kent J, Molony V, Robertson IS. Comparison of the Burdizzo and rubber ring methods for castrating and tail docking lambs. Vet Rec 1995;136:192–6.
9. Moloney V, Kent J, Robertson IS. Assessment of acute and chronic pain after different methods of castration in calves. Appl Anim Behav Sci 1995;46:33–48.
10. Flecknell PA. Analgesia and post-operative care. In: Laboratory animal anaesthesia. 3rd edition. London: Elsevier; 2009. p. 139–80.
11. Dubner R, Ren K. Assessing transient and persistent pain in animals. In: Wall PD, Melzack R, editors. Text book of pain. London: Harcourt; 1999. p. 359–69.
12. Roughan JV, Flecknell PA. Behavioural effects of laparotomy and analgesic effects of ketoprofen and carprofen in rats. Pain 2001;90:65–74.
13. Gross DR, Tranquilli WJ, Greene SA, et al. Critical anthropomorphic evaluation and treatment of postoperative pain in rats and mice. J Am Vet Med Assoc 2003;222:1505–10.
14. American College of Laboratory Animal Medicine. Public statement: recommendations for the assessment and management of pain in rabbits and rodents. J Am Assoc Lab Anim Sci 2007;46:97–108.

15. Miller AL. Detection and alleviation of pain and distress in laboratory rodents. PhD thesis, 2010.
16. Roughan JV, Flecknell PA. Evaluation of a short duration behaviour-based post-operative pain scoring system in rats. Eur J Pain 2003;7:397–406.
17. Roughan JV, Flecknell PA. Behaviour-based assessment of the duration of laparotomy-induced abdominal pain and the analgesic effects of carprofen and buprenorphine in rats. Behav Pharmacol 2004;15:461–72.
18. Wright-Williams SL. Behaviour-based assessment of post-operative pain in laboratory mice [PhD thesis] 2007.
19. Richardson CA, Flecknell PA. Anaesthesia and post-operative analgesia following experimental surgery in laboratory rodents: are we making progress? Altern Lab Anim 2005;33:119–27.
20. Dickinson AL, Leach MC, Flecknell PA. The analgesic effects of oral paracetamol in two strains of mice undergoing vasectomy. Lab Anim 2009;43:357–61.
21. Wright-Williams SL, Courade JP, Richardson CA, et al. Effects of vasectomy surgery and meloxicam treatment on faecal corticosterone and behaviour in two strains of laboratory mouse. Pain 2007;130:108–18.
22. Langford DJ, Bailey AL, Chanda ML, et al. Coding of facial expressions of pain in the laboratory mouse. Nat Methods 2010;7:447–52.
23. Svendson P. Pain expression in different laboratory animal species. Scand J Lab Anim Sci 1991;17:135–9.
24. Longley LA. Rodent anaesthesia. In: Anaesthesia of exotic pets. Edinburgh (Scotland): Elsevier; 2008. p. 59–84.
25. Roughan JV, Flecknell PA. Buprenorphine: a reappraisal of its antinociceptive effects and therapeutic use in alleviating post-operative pain in animals. Lab Anim 2002;36:322–43.
26. Aung HA, Mehendale SR, Xie JT, et al. Methylnaltrexone prevents morphine-induced kaolin intake in the rat. Life Sci 2004;74:2685–91.
27. Greenwood-Van Meerveld B, Gardner CJ, Little PJ, et al. Preclinical studies of opioids and opioid antagonists on gastrointestinal function. Neurogastroenterol Motil 2004;16(Suppl 2):46–53.
28. Jacobson C. Adverse effects on growth rates in rats caused by buprenorphine administration. Lab Anim 2000;34:202–6.
29. Committee for Veterinary Medicinal Products. Carprofen: summary report. EMEA/MRL/042/95-FINAL. Available at: http://www.ema.europa.eu/docs/en_GB/document_library/Maximum_Residue_Limits_-_Report/2009/11/WC500011412.pdf. Accessed August 5, 2010.
30. Julou L, Guyonnet C, Ducrot R, et al. Some pharmacological and toxicological studies on ketoprofen. Rheumatology 1976;15:5–10.
31. Lehmann HA, Baumeister M, Lützen L, et al. Meloxicam: a toxicology review. Inflammopharmacology 1996;4:105–23.
32. Wixson SK. Rabbits and rodents: anesthesia and analgesia. In: Hampshire V, Gonder JC. editors. Research animal anesthesia, analgesia and surgery. Greenbelt (MD): Scientists Center for Animal Welfare; 2007. p. 53–82.
33. Penderis J, Franklin RJ. Effects of pre- versus post-anaesthetic buprenorphine on propofol-anaesthetized rats. Vet Anaesth Analg 2005;32:256–60.
34. Criado AB, Gómez de Segura IA, Tendillo FJ, et al. Reduction of isoflurane MAC with buprenorphine and morphine in rats. Lab Anim 2000;34:252–9.
35. Hedenqvist P, Roughan JV, Flecknell PA. Effects of repeated anaesthesia with ketamine/medetomidine and of pre-anaesthetic administration of buprenorphine in rats. Lab Anim 2000;34:207–11.

36. Flecknell PA, Liles JH, Wiliamson HA. The use of lignocaine-prilocaine local anaesthetic cream for pain-free venepuncture in laboratory animals. Lab Anim 1990;24:142–6.
37. Lichtenberger M, Ko J. Anesthesia and analgesia for small mammals and birds. Veterinary Clinics of North America: Exotic Animal Practice; 2007;1:293–315.
38. Block BM, Liu SS, Rowlingson AJ, et al. Efficacy of postoperative epidural analgesia. JAMA 2003;290:2455–63.
39. Cheol Jin H, Keller AJ, Kwon Jung J, et al. Epidural tezampanel, an AMPA/kainate receptor antagonist, produces postoperative analgesia in rats. Anesth Analg 2007;105:1152–9.
40. Committee on Recognition and Alleviation of Pain in Laboratory Animals. Effective pain management. In: Recognition and alleviation of pain in laboratory animals. Washington, DC: National Academies Press; 2009. p. 71–118.
41. Franken ND, van Oostrom H, Stienen PJ, et al. Evaluation of analgesic and sedative effects of continuous infusion of dexemetomidine by measuring somatosensory- and auditory-evoked potentials in the rat. Vet Anaesth Analg 2008;35: 424–31.
42. De Matos R. Rodents: therapeutics. In: Keeble E, Meredith A, editors. BSAVA manual of rodents and ferrets. Gloucester (UK): BSAVA; 2009. p. 52–62.
43. Mogil JS. Animal models of pain: progress and challenges. Nat Rev Neurosci 2009;10:283–94.
44. Heard DJ. Anesthesia, analgesia and sedation of small mammals. In: Quesenberry KE, Carpenter JW, editors. Ferrets, rabbits and rodents clinical medicine and surgery. 2nd edition. Philadelphia: WB Saunders; 2000. p. 356–69.
45. Longley L. Anaesthesia and analgesia in rabbits and rodents. In Pract 2008;30: 92–7.
46. Hawkins MG. The use of analgesics in birds, reptiles and small exotic mammals. Journal of Exotic Pet Medicine 2006;15:177–92.

Rabbit Analgesia

Linda S. Barter, MVSc, PhD, DACVA

KEYWORDS

- Rabbit • Analgesia • Pain assessment • Opioid
- Nonsteroidal anti-inflammatory drugs

Rabbits are a very common household pet in the United States, with an estimated 6 million pet rabbits in 2007, an increase of almost 30% from 2001.[1] With increasing popularity, the complexity of diagnostic and surgical procedures performed on rabbits is increasing, along with the frequency of routine surgical procedures. More practitioners are faced with the need to provide adequate analgesia for this species. Pain is probably undertreated in animals in general and, at least in some parts of the world, it is less common to administer analgesics to rabbits as compared with dogs and cats.[2,3] Reasons for this may include less familiarity with the species, smaller knowledge base regarding analgesic dose, efficacy and safety in rabbits, concerns over possible side effects of some analgesics in rabbits, and the difficulties in assessing pain, and efficacy of pain management, in rabbits. While some of these concerns are valid, the underlying physiologic and anatomic similarities of all mammals would suggest that rabbits experience pain, like other more familiar mammalian species, and thus we are ethically obliged to provide relief to those animals in situations where it is likely they would experience pain such as trauma, surgery, and disease.

Untreated pain has many undesirable effects such as activation of complement cascade, cytokine systems, and arachidonic acid cascade, in addition to activation of the sympathetic nervous system. Sympathetic nervous system activation may result in tachycardia, arrhythmias, vasoconstriction, altered cardiac output, and increased myocardial oxygen demand. Alterations in organ perfusion, fluid, electrolyte, and acid-base balance may occur. Pain may alter respiratory rate and reduce tidal volume, which may intensify any existing respiratory compromise. Other detrimental effects of untreated pain include inducing a catabolic state, reduced appetite or anorexia, delayed wound healing, lowered immune responses, and prolonged hospital stays. Pain can also reduce gastrointestinal motility. Concurrent reductions in food intake, dehydration, and disease processes such as enterotoxemia and hepatic lipidosis, could all further promote ileus and may induce life-threatening problems in the rabbit. Critically ill or traumatized patients have the fewest physiologic reserves to deal with these additional insults. Untreated pain increases morbidity

The author has nothing to disclose.

Department of Surgical and Radiological Sciences, School of Veterinary Medicine, University of California, 2112 Tupper Hall, One Shields Avenue, Davis, CA 95616, USA

E-mail address: lsbarter@ucdavis.edu

Vet Clin Exot Anim 14 (2011) 93–104

doi:10.1016/j.cvex.2010.09.003

1094-9194/11/$ – see front matter. Published by Elsevier Inc.

and potentially increases mortality in many species, and maybe more so in a prey species like the rabbit. In the extreme, there are anecdotal reports of painful rabbits going into shock and dying despite their underlying illness or injury not appearing to have been life-threatening.

Understanding the physiology of pain is essential in the ability to prevent or alleviate pain. In simple terms, the pain pathway begins with detection of a noxious stimulus by the nervous system (transduction). This information is then relayed to the central nervous system (transmission) where information is integrated and processed and in turn relayed to higher centers, where it is interpreted as pain (perception). Analgesic drugs target the pain pathways at one or more of the aforementioned steps (multimodal analgesia). Untreated pain can increase the sensitivity of both the peripheral and central nervous system to stimuli, both painful and not traditionally considered painful, increasing the pain experienced by the animal or even creating scenarios whereby nonpainful stimuli, like touch, are painful to the animal. Persistent untreated pain may result in nervous system damage and the development of neuropathic pain. Although the evidence for such conditions in animals is sparse, neuropathic pain syndromes are being increasingly recognized in veterinary medicine.[4–6] Providing analgesia before application of the painful stimulus (preemptive analgesia prior to planned surgical interventions) may reduce nervous system changes in response to noxious input, as well as reduce postoperative pain levels and analgesic drug requirements. It is more difficult to control established pain. Perception is abolished by general anesthesia because those drugs produce unconsciousness, but many general anesthetics do not inhibit processing of noxious stimuli by the peripheral nervous system or spinal cord, and so do not prevent these aforementioned nervous system changes (sensitization). Concurrent administration of analgesic drugs to anesthetized patients undergoing painful procedures is warranted both pre- and intraoperatively as well as postoperatively. Heightened perception, for example by fear and/or anxiety, will likely increase pain perception and should be avoided. Pharmacologic treatment of pain is only part of a global pain management plan that also considers appropriate housing, husbandry, nursing care, physical therapy, and alternative therapeutic modalities such as acupuncture.

RECOGNIZING PAIN IN RABBITS

Recognizing pain in any species can be challenging but particularly so in the rabbit. There are no generally accepted objective criteria for assessing the degree of pain experienced by a rabbit, and individuals can vary greatly in their response to painful stimuli. In other companion species, behavior-based pain scoring systems have been developed and implemented with success in clinical practice.[7,8] Behavior-based pain assessment schemes are those that include assessment of behaviors and interaction with the animal. Attempts have been made to develop such systems in rabbits but with little success, due to the effects of the observer on animal behavior.[9] There are also several contributory factors. As a prey species, rabbits evolved to hide weaknesses to avoid predation, and as such they may hide their pain to keep a normal appearance when directly observed by strangers. Normal rabbits are bright, alert, active, and very inquisitive; however, an anxious or scared rabbit will freeze and thus its behavior is not assessable. Clinically, rabbits often appear to respond to pain or distress by remaining motionless and so have little activity or behavior to be assessed. To exhibit normal behavior it is important that rabbits be housed in an environment in which they feel safe. In addition, behavioral observations by strangers may need to be made indirectly through a viewing panel or camera in order for the animals to behave freely.[10] Behavioral observations are best made by individuals with detailed knowledge of normal rabbit behavior in given situations, and ideally the behavior of the individual rabbit.

Alterations in heart rate, respiratory rate, and blood pressure may be consistent with pain but these can also be caused by a variety of other factors. These parameters are under complex physiologic control and may be altered by pharmacologic agents, disease processes, stress, and anxiety (and it is likely that any hospitalized, sick, or injured rabbit will be anxious). Restraint has been shown to alter physiologic parameters such as respiratory and heart rate.[11] Changes in heart rate and respiratory rate in dogs have been shown not to correlate with pain scores.[12] More sophisticated evaluation of heart rate variability may be more indicative of pain; however, this is not within the realms of clinical medicine at this time.[13,14]

Animals in pain frequently reduce their food and water intake, or stop eating and drinking altogether, resulting in weight loss and anorexia associated with gastrointestinal problems. Appetite and weight changes have been used as indicators of pain.[15–17] In laboratory rabbits after ovariohysterectomy, food and water consumption was reduced for 2 to 3 days after surgery and was associated with significant reduction in body weight.[10] Although the evidence is consistent that pain reduces food and water intake, pain is not the only potential cause and therefore these signs are not specific. In addition, such changes are typically only apparent in retrospect, and may not be useful in assessing an animal in acute pain.

Behavioral indicators of pain include changes in posture, locomotion, or gait. Posture is altered to avoid moving or contacting painful areas of the body (guarding) and locomotor activity is reduced overall.[18] In laboratory studies, rabbits with acute foot pain had sudden movements and vocalizing, followed by limping, abnormal posture, and licking of the affected area.[19] In these group-housed animals, both social and motor activity of the affected animals was significantly reduced. Of note, the behavior of the entire group was affected by pain in the dominant member of the group. Pain in a member of a group of rabbits may be one factor to evaluate if changes in group dynamics occur.

The effect of pain on activity levels may also depend on the time of day and the intensity of the stimulus.[20] Acclimatized laboratory rabbits were videotaped pre- and post-ovariohysterectomy, and their behavior analyzed to compile several behaviors that may be useful indicators of pain in rabbits.[10] In this study "inactive pain behavior" was considered the most useful indicator of pain, as it was observed either not at all or very infrequently preoperatively, and very frequently postoperatively. In further support of such behaviors as indicators of pain, they decreased in frequency during each of the 4 postoperative days. Inactive pain behaviors consisted of twitching (rapid fur movement on the back), wincing (rapid backward movement associated with eye closing and swallowing), staggering (partial loss of balance), flinching (rapid upward body jerks for no reason), pressing (pushing abdomen toward floor), very slow postural adjustments, and shuffling (walking at very slow pace).

In the aforementioned study, behaviors that indicate activity (movement, searching, interaction, rearing, standing, grooming, and exploring) decreased, and behaviors that indicate inactivity (no-behavior, lying down) increased immediately postoperatively compared with preoperative values, and did not return to baseline for 3 days.[10] Activity behaviors, either reduced activity or increased inactivity, may be challenging to use for assessment of pain in rabbits because there is considerable variation between individuals and it requires long periods of indirect observation. In addition, in the ovariohysterectomy study rabbits were significantly more active in the afternoon than in the morning, and there was considerable variation between individuals.[10] Moreover, long periods and indirect observation are required to assess changes in the duration of those behaviors. Other problems with using activity type behaviors are considering how those behaviors will be affected by drugs, for example, sedation or anesthetic recovery, or disease (systemic debilitation) that may preclude the animal from moving or exploring and yet not always be associated with pain.

NONPHARMACOLOGIC CONSIDERATIONS FOR PAIN MANAGEMENT

Factors other than drug therapy should not be overlooked in pain management in rabbits. Gentle tissue handling and good surgical technique will reduce the degree of postoperative pain. While hospitalized, rabbits should be provided with appropriate housing that is away from the sight, smell, and sound of predatory species. The area should be quiet and the animals kept clean and dry. Attention should be paid to making sure animals have easy access to food and water, particularly if they have mobility issues. Appropriate nursing care by attending to wounds, bandages, urination, and defecation will also help to improve patient comfort. Animals should be handled carefully and restrained appropriately to avoid unnecessary stress. Some animals that are normally housed with another rabbit may find the social isolation stressful, and consideration should be given to bringing their "buddy" rabbit into hospital with them.

PHARMACOLOGIC PAIN MANAGEMENT

Acute pain can occur following surgical procedures, trauma, and a variety of medical conditions, particularly those associated with an inflammatory component. To create an analgesic plan it is helpful to consider the pain severity, likely duration, whether the animal will be hospitalized, and the level of monitoring and care available. Drugs can then be selected to address those criteria in conjunction with factors such as underlying medical or physiologic conditions that may increase an animal's susceptibility to side effects of some classes of drugs.

There are 5 main classes of drugs used for acute pain management: opioids, nonsteroidal anti-inflammatory drugs (NSAIDs), local anesthetics, α2-agonists, and miscellaneous (eg, N-methyl-D-aspartate [NMDA] receptor antagonists, serotonin reuptake inhibitors, calcium channel antagonists). There is comparatively little experimental work published on analgesics in rabbits. Most of the drugs and doses used in practice today are based on extrapolation from other species and clinical experience. Suggested doses and routes of administration of analgesic drugs for use in the rabbit are listed in **Table 1**.

Opioids

Opioids are the mainstay for management of moderate to severe pain. Opioids produce analgesia by binding to mu and/or kappa opioid receptors. These receptors are found within the central nervous system, where they exert antinociceptive effects by inhibiting ascending nociceptive input, activating descending inhibitory pathways, and decreasing neurotransmitter release.[21] A growing body of work suggests that opioids may also act peripherally in inflamed tissues.[22] These drugs can be administered systemically, orally, locally (eg, intra-articular), and via the epidural or subarachnoid route. Significant opioid side effects in mammals include sedation, respiratory depression, and reduced gastrointestinal motility. The inhibition of gastrointestinal peristalsis is due to activation of mu and/or kappa opioid receptors expressed by enteric neurons and intestinal muscle cells.[23] Both mu and kappa opioid receptor agonists have been shown experimentally to inhibit motility in the isolated rabbit

Table 1
Suggested systemic analgesic drugs and dosages for use in rabbits[a]

Drug	Dose (mg/kg)	Route	Interval (hours)	References	Comments
Opioids					
Buprenorphine	0.02–0.1	SQ, IM, IV	6	[27]	Reported duration of effect variable and may be dose dependent, clinical duration may only be 4–6 h
Butorphanol	0.1–0.5	SQ, IM, IV	2	[27,28]	Duration of effect may be dose dependent
Morphine	2.0–5.0	SQ, IM	3–4	[31]	
	0.1	Epidurally		[a]	
Oxymorphone	0.1–0.3	SQ, IM, IV	3–4	[a]	
Tramadol	10	PO	12–24	[a]	Pharmacokinetic data reported to be variable, data on clinical efficacy lacking
NSAIDs					
Carprofen	4.0	SQ	24	[a]	
	2.0–4.0	PO	12–24	[a]	
Meloxicam	0.3–0.5	SQ	24	[a]	
	0.5–1.5	PO	24	[10,38]	

Abbreviations: IM, intramuscular; IV, intravenous; PO, per os (orally); SQ, subcutaneous.
[a] Recommendation based on personal experience and anecdotal reports.

intestine.[24,25] Morphine administered intrathecally to rabbits has been shown to suppress duodenal peristalsis.[26]

The analgesic efficacy of systemically administered opioids has been evaluated in some experimental models of pain in rabbits. Buprenorphine, butorphanol, nalbuphine, and pentazocine all increased skin twitch latency in response to focused laser applied to the shaved dorsum of experimental rabbits.[27] In that study, increasing doses of buprenorphine from 0.0075 mg/kg to 0.3 mg/kg appeared to have little effect on maximum analgesia (as assessed by prolongation of skin twitch), but did increase duration of effects from an average of 150 minutes at the lowest dose to greater than 780 minutes at the highest dose. This finding is consistent with the agonist-antagonist (eg, butorphanol) or partial-agonist opioids (buprenorphine) displaying a "ceiling effect" in the magnitude of analgesia they provide.[21] Due to this ceiling effect, opioids of this category are suitable for the treatment of mild to moderate pain. In addition, the half-life of butorphanol in the rabbit is short, and duration of effect is limited to 2 to 3 hours at maximum.[27,28]

Buprenorphine is one of the most commonly used opioids in rabbits because of to its long duration of effect, as well as its partial-agonist activity and assumed lower incidence of side effects compared with mu-agonist opioids. Experimental evidence to support this is limited. Buprenorphine has been documented to reduce respiratory rate, slightly increase arterial pCO_2 levels, and produce mild hypoxemia in awake healthy rabbits at a dose of 0.016 to 0.02 mg/kg administered intravenously.[29] Despite limited experimental evidence suggesting a duration of effects of over 12 hours, clinically the duration of analgesic provided by buprenorphine is variable and may last only up to 6 hours.[27]

Buprenorphine should be reserved for the management of mild to moderate pain that is not expected to change in severity. First, due to its limited analgesic potency, increasing doses are not likely to increase the magnitude of analgesia. The behavioral signs of pain associated with experimental myoma viral infection were not abrogated by buprenorphine at 0.03 mg/kg every 12 hours.[30] Second, buprenorphine has a high affinity for mu opioid receptors and, as such, is hard to displace from those receptors, either by an antagonist if reversal is desired or by a pure agonist if more potent analgesia is required.

Mu opioid receptor agonists are the most effective therapy for acute pain, providing rapid-onset, dose-dependent analgesia. Morphine has been shown to be an effective analgesic in rabbits in a thermal stimulus based experimental model.[31] Other mu-agonists such as oxymorphone and hydromorphone have been reported anecdotally to be effective analgesics in rabbits, with fewer side effects than morphine. In many species, there is marked individual variation in dose requirements, side effects, and tolerance to opioids of the same class; this is likely also true in rabbits. Although rabbits should be monitored for undesirable effects of opioids, pain in itself can also result in respiratory depression, abnormal behavior, depressed food intake, and ileus. Concern regarding those effects should not result in the withholding of adequate analgesia to painful rabbits. Opioid-associated ileus needs to be identified early, and managed by syringe feeding and by maintaining adequate hydration.

Opioids may cause sedation in rabbits. Whereas buprenorphine does not cause obvious reduction in activity levels in healthy rabbits, butorphanol and the mu-agonist opioids can cause marked reductions in activity levels and moderate to marked sedation, particularly at high doses.[27,31] The magnitude of sedation or inactivity produced by opioids may be affected by systemic health of the individual rabbit and its level of pain, and these factors should be considered when evaluating the therapeutic efficacy.

Fentanyl is a potent mu opioid receptor agonist with short duration of action, used commonly in combination with fluanisone as an anesthetic premedicant in rabbits in some parts of the world.[32,33] In other species fentanyl is most commonly used as an infusion during anesthesia or in the immediate postoperative period to provide titratable, potent analgesia. Fentanyl constant-rate infusions have been used intraoperatively to provide analgesia to rabbits and subjectively allow lowering of anesthetic vaporizer settings. However, respiratory depression at higher doses can be marked, necessitating positive pressure ventilation. Dose requirements, efficacy, anesthetic sparing, and hemodynamic effects vary between species and have not been reported in rabbits.

Transdermally delivered fentanyl results in variable plasma levels in rabbits.[34] In some rabbits rapid hair regrowth in the patch application area was thought to significantly inhibit drug absorption. Twelve to 24 hours after application of a 25 μg/h patch, average plasma fentanyl concentrations ranged from 0.5 to 1.5 ng/mL and remained there until patch removal at 72 hours. Interindividual variation was marked and, although those plasma levels would be considered therapeutic in people, the therapeutic plasma fentanyl concentration required for analgesia in the rabbit is not known.

Morphine, due to its intermediate lipid solubility, is well suited for epidural administration. Onset of effect is slow (up to 1 hour); however, systemic uptake is limited and the duration of effect is long (up to 20 hours in some species). Epidural administration of preservative-free morphine may be useful for perioperative analgesia in rabbits undergoing orthopedic surgery or extensive surgery of the abdominal or thoracic cavities, with minimal systemic effects and no motor blockade. The lumbosacral epidural injection technique in rabbits is similar to that described for other small animal species, with the exceptions of the interarcuate ligament not being very deep and a distinct "pop" not often being perceived when passing through it.[35] The rabbit spinal cord terminates within the sacral vertebrae, typically at the level of S2.[36] The incidence of subarachnoid puncture is relatively high in rabbits when epidural puncture is attempted, because of these anatomic features. In such circumstances cerebrospinal fluid either appears in the hub of the needle or can be aspirated. One-third to one-half of the drug dose and volume calculated for epidural administration can be administered into the subarachnoid space.

Nonsteroidal Anti-Inflammatory Drugs

As a group, these drugs have anti-inflammatory, analgesic, and antipyretic activity, and are useful for management of mild to moderate acute or chronic pain, particularly if there is an inflammatory component.[37] These agents appear to act synergistically with opioids, such that lower doses of opioids can be used in combination with NSAIDs. Onset of action of NSAIDs is relatively slow and the dosing interval relatively long. Oral NSAIDs are particularly useful for extending postoperative pain control for several days and in managing chronically painful conditions. These drugs have well known side effects in other species including renal dysfunction, hepatic dysfunction, gastrointestinal ulceration, and inhibition of platelet function. Although theoretically these drugs would seem to be most beneficial when administered before tissue injury, their use preoperatively remains controversial due to their potential for harm. Even healthy rabbits are frequently hypotensive under general anesthesia, which may increase the risk for development of side effects from these drugs. The clinical significance of this has not been well investigated in the rabbit.

NSAIDs have been used extensively in rabbits, although there is little published information. The pharmacokinetics of orally administered meloxicam, a cyclooxygenase-2 preferential NSAID, has been reported.[38] In this study significant interindividual variability in absorption and clearance was reported. There were no obvious adverse clinical effects, changes in serum biochemistry, or deviations in normal weight gain in healthy New Zealand white rabbits after daily administration of 1.5 mg/kg for 5 days. Oral administration of meloxicam is well tolerated by rabbits.[10,38] Meloxicam per os at 1 mg/kg post surgery followed by 0.5 mg/kg once daily for the 2 following days caused a significant reduction in some pain-associated behaviors associated with ovariohysterectomy.[10] Due to the side effect profile of NSAIDs in other species, consideration should be given to monitoring rabbits receiving chronic NSAID therapy with serum biochemistry profiles and fecal occult blood tests.

Local Anesthetics

Local anesthetics, such as lidocaine and bupivacaine, are used commonly in veterinary medicine to reversibly inhibit neural transmission. Local anesthetics can be applied topically, via infiltration, administered intra-articularly, by regional nerve block, or by epidural or subarachnoid injection. Analgesia to the desensitized area is complete and, by abolishing neural input to the central nervous system, the immediate central sensitization induced by noxious stimulation is reduced. Local anesthetic techniques can be useful in conjunction with general anesthesia to provide analgesia, reduce the required anesthetic dose, and reduce postoperative analgesic requirements.

Incisional line blocks and wound infiltration are simple, cost-effective means to provide analgesia that are underutilized in small animal medicine. Doses of 2 mg/kg lidocaine and 1 mg/kg bupivacaine would be suitable for such purposes. Specific nerve blocks may be particularly useful to facilitate dental procedures in rabbits. Directions for performing infraorbital, mental, mandibular, and maxillary nerve blocks have been described in the rabbit.[39]

Epidural or subarachnoid administration of local anesthetic can be performed in the rabbit, resulting in complete sensory and mild to severe motor impairment to the hind limbs. Epidural administration of 0.2 mL/kg of 2% lidocaine results in rapid-onset (1–3 minutes) sensory and motor block to the hind-quarters of approximately 30 to 40 minutes' duration in rabbits.[40] Bupivacaine is longer lasting and, if used at lower concentrations, may produce a more discriminative block, providing longer epidural analgesia with minimal motor effects. Bupivacaine has not been well investigated in rabbits. In practical terms, hind-limb motor blockade in nonanesthetized rabbits may cause them severe distress and lead to self-induced injury. Considerations and side effects of epidural or subarachnoid local anesthetics are the same as those in other species.

Intravenous infusion of lidocaine has become popular recently for provision of analgesia and as a gastrointestinal promotility agent in other species. The clinical use of lidocaine for this purpose has not been investigated in the rabbit. In the cat, lidocaine infusion has a significant negative impact on the cardiovascular system[41]; however, there is some evidence to suggest that this is not the case in rabbits.[42] Further investigations on efficacy and safety are warranted before lidocaine infusions can be recommended for analgesia in rabbits.

Local anesthetics have dose-related toxic side effects on both the central nervous system and the cardiovascular system. Care should be taken to avoid administration of toxic doses of local anesthetics in small patients such as rabbits. Although not well documented, doses of bupivacaine and lidocaine below 2 and 4 mg/kg, respectively, for infiltration or regional block, should avoid toxicosis.

α2-Adrenergic Agonists

The α2-adrenergic agonists possess sedative, muscle relaxant, sympatholytic, and analgesic properties, and are reversible. Used pre- or intraoperatively they can also dramatically reduce anesthetic requirements.[43] These drugs have a marked impact on the cardiovascular system, reducing heart rate and cardiac output. Their use should be reserved for clinically healthy patients. "Microdose" medetomidine has been suggested to avoid the negative cardiovascular effects of these drugs, and although the magnitude of cardiovascular depression is dose dependent, even small doses produce clinically relevant reductions in cardiac output. In the dog, 1 μg/kg reduced cardiac index by greater than 50% of baseline,[44] and constant-rate infusions of 1, 2, and 3 μg/kg/h reduced cardiac index by 50%, 65%, and 70%, respectively, from baseline.[45]

Miscellaneous Drugs

The NMDA receptor antagonist ketamine is used commonly in rabbits for heavy sedation to anesthesia. The NMDA receptor has a significant role in the development of central sensitization. NMDA receptor antagonism may reduce this phenomenon and thus reduce postoperative analgesic requirements.[46] Ketamine infusions have been suggested in veterinary patients as having anesthetic-sparing and antihyperalgesic effects; however, these have not been studied in rabbits. NMDA receptor antagonists have also been used with some success in rodent models of chronic pain.[47] The psychomimetic, sedative, and motor effects of higher doses of ketamine limit its use for such purposes; however, other NMDA receptor antagonists devoid of those properties may be useful. Clinically, chronic pain syndromes have not been well recognized to date in the rabbit; however, as our understanding and ability to recognize pain in rabbits increases, such syndromes are likely to become apparent.

Tramadol is an analgesic with multiple mechanisms of action. Tramadol has some activity as a mu opioid receptor agonist; it also has serotonin and norepinephrine reuptake inhibitory activity and α2-adrenergic agonist activity.[21] The pharmacokinetics of tramadol have been described in the rabbit after both oral and intravenous administration.[48,49] Intravenous administration of tramadol in isoflurane-anesthetized rabbits resulted in widely variable plasma levels of tramadol and its M1 metabolite.[50] After oral administration of 11 mg/kg of tramadol, plasma concentration of tramadol and its active metabolite O-desmethyltramadol (M1) were variable and below those levels considered analgesic in people.[49] Therapeutic plasma levels in the rabbit are not known, and the effective dose and dosing interval have not been established in rabbits. Tramadol anecdotally has been used in the clinical management of chronic pain in rabbits; however, palatability appears to be an issue when compounding the drug for use in rabbits.

SUMMARY

Due to their evolution as a prey species, rabbits are reluctant to demonstrate abnormal behavior in the presence of an observer and as such are a challenging species in which to identify pain. Creation of a rabbit-friendly environment within the veterinary hospital in conjunction with remote observation will facilitate detection of behaviors commonly associated with pain, such as reduced activity, reduced motility, abnormal posture, wincing, flinching, abdominal pressing, and staggering. An effective analgesic plan has both pharmacologic and nonpharmacologic components. Analgesic therapy should target multiple locations within the pain pathway, and is an integral part of the management of surgical and trauma patients as well as acute and chronic medical conditions in the rabbit. Many analgesics are associated with side effects; however, with careful dosing and monitoring these are unlikely to be as detrimental to the patient as untreated pain.

REFERENCES

1. American Veterinary Medical Association. U.S. Pet Ownership & Demographics Sourcebook (2007 Edition). 2007. Available at: http://www.avma.org/reference/marketstats/sourcebook.asp. Accessed September 14, 2010.
2. Lascelles BD, Capner CA, Waterman-Pearson AE. Current British attitudes to perioperative analgesia for cats and small mammals. Vet Rec 1999;145:601–4.
3. Capner CA, Lascelles BD, Waterman-Pearson AE. Current British veterinary attitudes to perioperative analgesia for dogs. Vet Rec 1999;145(4):95–9.
4. O'Hagan BJ. Neuropathic pain in a cat post-amputation. Aust Vet J 2006;84(3): 83–6.
5. Muir WW 3rd, Wiese AJ, Wittum TE. Prevalence and characteristics of pain in dogs and cats examined as outpatients at a veterinary teaching hospital. J Am Vet Med Assoc 2004;224(9):1459–63.
6. Shaver SL, Robinson NG, Wright BD, et al. A multimodal approach to management of suspected neuropathic pain in a prairie falcon (Falco mexicanus). J Avian Med Surg 2009;23(3):209–13.
7. Holton L, Reid J, Scott EM, et al. Development of a behaviour-based scale to measure acute pain in dogs. Vet Rec 2001;148(17):525–31.

8. Murrell JC, Psatha EP, Scott EM, et al. Application of a modified form of the Glasgow pain scale in a veterinary teaching centre in the Netherlands. Vet Rec 2008; 162(13):403–8.
9. Roughan JV, Flecknell PA, Orr H. Behavioral assessment of post-operative pain and analgesic effects of carprofen in the domestic rabbit. Abstracts presented at: the World Congress of Veterinary Anesthesia. Knoxville (TN), 17–20 September, 2003. Vet Anaesth Analg 2004;31:282–91.
10. Leach MC, Allweiler S, Richardson C, et al. Behavioural effects of ovariohysterectomy and oral administration of meloxicam in laboratory housed rabbits. Res Vet Sci 2009;87(2):336–47.
11. MeEwen GN Jr. Thermoregulatory responses of restrained versus unrestrained rabbits. Life Sci 1975;17(6):901–5.
12. Holton LL, Scott EM, Nolan AM, et al. Relationship between physiological factors and clinical pain in dogs scored using a numerical rating scale. J Small Anim Pract 1998;39(10):469–74.
13. Arras M, Rettich A, Cinelli P, et al. Assessment of post-laparotomy pain in laboratory mice by telemetric recording of heart rate and heart rate variability. BMC Vet Res 2007;3:16.
14. Rietmann TR, Stauffacher M, Bernasconi P, et al. The association between heart rate, heart rate variability, endocrine and behavioural pain measures in horses suffering from laminitis. J Vet Med A Physiol Pathol Clin Med 2004; 51(5):218–25.
15. Wheat NJ, Cooper DM. A simple method for assessing analgesic requirements and efficacy in rodents. Lab Anim (NY) 2009;38(7):246–7.
16. Shavit Y, Fish G, Wolf G, et al. The effects of perioperative pain management techniques on food consumption and body weight after laparotomy in rats. Anesth Analg 2005;101(4):1112–6 [table of contents].
17. Liles JH, Flecknell PA. The effects of buprenorphine, nalbuphine and butorphanol alone or following halothane anaesthesia on food and water consumption and locomotor movement in rats. Lab Anim 1992;26(3):180–9.
18. Flecknell PA, Morton DB. Use of animals in research. Vet Rec 1991;128(22):531.
19. Farabollini F, Giordano G, Carli G. Tonic pain and social behavior in male rabbits. Behav Brain Res 1988;31(2):169–75.
20. Aloisi AM, Lupo C, Carli G. Effects of formalin-induced pain on exploratory behaviour in rabbits. Neuroreport 1993;4(6):739–42.
21. Gutstein HB, Akil H. Chapter 21. Opioid analgesics. In: Brunton LL, Lazo JS, Parker KL, editors. Goodman & Gilman's the pharmacological basis of therapeutics. 11th edition. New York (NY): McGraw-Hill Companies; 2010. p. 547–90.
22. Stein C, Lang LJ. Peripheral mechanisms of opioid analgesia. Curr Opin Pharmacol 2009;9(1):3–8.
23. Shahbazian A, Heinemann A, Schmidhammer H, et al. Involvement of mu- and kappa-, but not delta-, opioid receptors in the peristaltic motor depression caused by endogenous and exogenous opioids in the guinea-pig intestine. Br J Pharmacol 2002;135(3):741–50.
24. Cosola C, Albrizio M, Guaricci AC, et al. Opioid agonist/antagonist effect of naloxone in modulating rabbit jejunum contractility in vitro. J Physiol Pharmacol 2006;57(3):439–49.
25. Nomura Y, Hayashi S. Pre- and post-synaptic effects of spiradoline and U-50488H, selective kappa opioid receptor agonists, in isolated ileum. Scand J Gastroenterol 1992;27(4):295–302.

26. Dai JL, Ren ZJ, Fu ZM, et al. Electroacupuncture reversed the inhibition of intestinal peristalsis induced by intrathecal injection of morphine in rabbits. Chin Med J (Engl) 1993;106(3):220–4.

27. Flecknell PA, Liles JH. Assessment of the analgesic action of opioid agonist-antagonists in the rabbit. J Assoc Vet Anaesthetics 1990;17:24–9.

28. Portnoy LG, Hustead DR. Pharmacokinetics of butorphanol tartrate in rabbits. Am J Vet Res 1992;53(4):541–3.

29. Shafford HL, Schadt JC. Respiratory and cardiovascular effects of buprenorphine in conscious rabbits. Vet Anaesth Analg 2008;35(4):326–32.

30. Robinson AJ, Muller WJ, Braid AL, et al. The effect of buprenorphine on the course of disease in laboratory rabbits infected with myxoma virus. Lab Anim 1999;33(3):252–7.

31. Barter LS, Kwaitkowski AE. Thermal threshold testing for evaluation of analgesics in rabbits. Paper presented at: Annual Meeting American College of Veterinary Anesthesiologists. Chicago (IL), September 10, 2009.

32. Flecknell PA, John M, Mitchell M, et al. Neuroleptanalgesia in the rabbit. Lab Anim 1983;17(2):104–9.

33. Martinez MA, Murison PJ, Love E. Induction of anaesthesia with either midazolam or propofol in rabbits premedicated with fentanyl/fluanisone. Vet Rec 2009; 164(26):803–6.

34. Foley PL, Henderson AL, Bissonette EA, et al. Evaluation of fentanyl transdermal patches in rabbits: blood concentrations and physiologic response. Comp Med 2001;51(3):239–44.

35. Skarda RT, Tranquilli WJ. Local and regional anesthetic and analgesic techniques: cats. In: Tranquilli WJ, Thurmon JC, Grimm KA, editors. Lumb & Jones' veterinary anesthesia and analgesia. 4th edition. Ames (IA): Blackwell Publishing; 2007. p. 595–603.

36. Greenaway JB, Partlow GD, Gonsholt NL, et al. Anatomy of the lumbosacral spinal cord in rabbits. J Am Anim Hosp Assoc 2001;37(1):27–34.

37. Burke A, Smyth E, FitzGerald GA. Chapter 26. Analgesic-antipyretic and antiinflammatory agents; pharmacotherapy of gout. In: Brunton LL, Lazo JS, Parker KL, editors. Goodman & Gilman's the pharmacological basis of therapeutics. 11th edition. New York (NY): McGraw-Hill Companies; 2010.

38. Turner PV, Chen HC, Taylor WM. Pharmacokinetics of meloxicam in rabbits after single and repeat oral dosing. Comp Med 2006;56(1):63–7.

39. Lichtenberger M, Ko J. Anesthesia and analgesia for small mammals and birds. Vet Clin North Am Exot Anim Pract 2007;10(2):293–315.

40. Doherty MM, Hughes PJ, Korszniak NV, et al. Prolongation of lidocaine-induced epidural anesthesia by medium molecular weight hyaluronic acid formulations: pharmacodynamic and pharmacokinetic studies in the rabbit. Anesth Analg 1995;80(4):740–6.

41. Pypendop BH, Ilkiw JE. Assessment of the hemodynamic effects of lidocaine administered IV in isoflurane-anesthetized cats. Am J Vet Res 2005;66(4):661–8.

42. Taniguchi T, Shibata K, Yamamoto K, et al. Effects of lidocaine administration on hemodynamics and cytokine responses to endotoxemia in rabbits. Crit Care Med 2000;28(3):755–9.

43. Grint NJ, Murison PJ. A comparison of ketamine-midazolam and ketamine-medetomidine combinations for induction of anaesthesia in rabbits. Vet Anaesth Analg 2008;35(2):113–21.

44. Pypendop BH, Verstegen JP. Hemodynamic effects of medetomidine in the dog: a dose titration study. Vet Surg 1998;27(6):612–22.

45. Carter JE, Campbell NB, Posner LP, et al. The hemodynamic effects of medeto-midine continuous rate infusions in the dog. Vet Anaesth Analg 2010;37(3): 197–206.

46. Suzuki M. Role of N-methyl-D-aspartate receptor antagonists in postoperative pain management. Curr Opin Anaesthesiol 2009;22(5):618–22.

47. Holtman JR Jr, Crooks PA, Johnson-Hardy JK, et al. Effects of norketamine enan-tiomers in rodent models of persistent pain. Pharmacol Biochem Behav 2008; 90(4):676–85.

48. Kucuk A, Kadioglu Y, Celebi F. Investigation of the pharmacokinetics and deter-mination of tramadol in rabbit plasma by a high-performance liquid chromatog-raphy-diode array detector method using liquid-liquid extraction. J Chromatogr B Analyt Technol Biomed Life Sci 2005;816(1–2):203–8.

49. Souza MJ, Greenacre CB, Cox SK. Pharmacokinetics of orally administered tra-madol in domestic rabbits (Oryctolagus cuniculus). Am J Vet Res 2008;69(8): 979–82.

50. Egger CM, Souza MJ, Greenacre CB, et al. Effect of intravenous administration of tramadol hydrochloride on the minimum alveolar concentration of isoflurane in rabbits. Am J Vet Res 2009;70(8):945–9.

Pain Management in Ferrets

Hugo van Oostrom, DVM, PhD*,
Nico J. Schoemaker, DVM, PhD, DECZM (small mammal & avian), DABVP (Avian),
Joost J. Uilenreef, DVM, MVR, DECVAA

KEYWORDS

• Pain • Ferret • Nonsteroidal anti-inflammatory drugs • Opioids

Along with the growing popularity of ferrets as pets comes the demand for advanced veterinary care for these patients. The number of ferrets brought to the veterinarian has steadily increased and might increase even further over the coming years. Among these ferrets are individuals experiencing a painful condition. Pain is associated with a broad range of conditions, including acute or chronic inflammatory disease, neoplasia, and trauma, as well as iatrogenic causes, such as surgery and diagnostic procedures. Pain should be treated from a welfare, ethical, and medical perspective. It is well documented that poor pain management in the postoperative period has detrimental effects on recovery, including wound healing and maximal restoration of function of the patient.[1,2]

Effective pain management requires knowledge and skills to assess pain, good understanding of the pathophysiology of pain, and general knowledge of pharmacologic and pharmacodynamic principles. Veterinarians also need to consider species-specific issues and requirements regarding the aforementioned items. Unfortunately, scientific studies on efficacy, pharmacokinetics, pharmacodynamics, and safety of analgesic drugs in the ferret are limited. However, basic rules in the treatment of pain and on mechanisms of action, safety, and efficacy of analgesic drugs in other species can be adapted and applied to pain management in ferrets.

This article aims to make an inventory of what is known on the recognition of pain in ferrets, what analgesic drugs are currently used in ferrets, and how they can be adopted in a patient-orientated pain management plan to provide effective pain relief while reducing and monitoring for unwanted side effects.

RECOGNIZING PAIN

One should be able to recognize pain to treat it. Recognizing pain in animals is difficult, primarily because of the lack of verbal communication. In veterinary medicine, it is well

Department of Clinical Sciences of Companion Animals, Faculty of Veterinary Medicine, Utrecht University, PO Box 80.154 NL-3508 TD Utrecht, The Netherlands
* Corresponding author.
E-mail address: h.vanoostrom@uu.nl

Vet Clin Exot Anim 14 (2011) 105–116
doi:10.1016/j.cvex.2010.09.001
1094-9194/11/$ – see front matter © 2011 Elsevier Inc. All rights reserved.

vetexotic.theclinics.com

known that different species express pain in different ways. There is a strong supposition that solitary-living animals and prey animals are masters of disguising pain. Different forms of pain might induce different types of pain-related behaviors, complicating the recognition of pain even more. Therefore, pain scales should include behavioral parameters that are species-specific, can be objectively assessed, and indicate different forms of pain, for example, pain due to trauma, acute postoperative pain, pain from the musculoskeletal system, visceral pain, and inflammatory pain.

Although ferrets are used as laboratory models in neurophysiologic studies, including studies involving nociception and pain,[3–9] most of these studies do not report on the behavioral changes potentially related to nociception and pain.

To determine specific behavioral signs of pain in ferrets, one should get familiar with the normal behavior of this species first.[10,11] Flecknell[10] stresses the need for taking the time to adequately observe the animal to assess whether it is in pain or not. Making adequate assessments in ferrets may therefore be impaired by their normal activity levels, because they spend up to 70% of their time per day sleeping, with short episodes of activity in between.[12,13] Therefore, waiting for the ferret to be awake and display active behavior is recommended for making a sound assessment of the animal. Behavioral characteristics that are frequently seen in animals with pain are (1) diminished general activity and exploratory behavior in a new environment; (2) altered posture (in many animals, a hunched posture but in ferrets, the normal hunchback is now absent); (3) altered gait, such as lameness; (4) uncharacteristic aggression in animals that are otherwise very friendly; (5) apathy in animals that are otherwise fierce; (6) vocalizations that differ in pitch and pattern from the normal interactive sounds; (7) hiding in the back of the cage facing away from the observer; (8) lack of grooming behavior resulting in ruffled and unkempt appearance of the hair coat; (9) diminished food and water intake, especially in dental or gastrointestinal pain; (10) bruxism, especially in abdominal pain; and (11) aversive response to external palpation of the animal.

A gross subset of behavioral signs of pain in the ferret has been described in clinical reviews.[14,15] The signs included anorexia, lethargy, crying, stiff movements, inability to curl into a sleeping position, and squinting; however, these reports did not mention whether and how the clinical validity of these parameters was established. Johnston[11] describes some specific pain-related behaviors that he encountered as a clinician working with ferrets. These behaviors include inactivity, staying curled in a ball (opposed to what Brown[14] and Pollock[15] reported), aggression, teeth-baring when being disturbed, decreased appetite, shivering when body temperature is normal, bristling of the tail fur, half-closed eyelids, focal muscle fasciculations, high-pitched vocalization or grunting when handled, lameness, and general malaise. Behavioral parameters of pain in ferrets described by Lichtenberger and Ko[16] include depression, immobility, silent demeanor, distanced from their environment, half-closed eyes, lack of grooming behavior, bruxism, and hiding themselves.

Sladky and colleagues[17] describe behavioral parameters of pain in ferrets in a study on the effectiveness of epidural morphine for postoperative analgesia after ovariohysterectomy and anal sacculectomy. The authors adapted a pain scale used in scoring pain in dogs after ovariohysterectomy by Hardie and colleagues.[18] Also, an ethogram of different behavioral parameters was made to extract possible pain-related behaviors. Although the number of animals in the control and treatment group was small and the duration of behavior assessed was short, a few behavioral parameters were suggested to be related to pain. These parameters were restricted/labored respiratory patterns, trembling, and attenuation of movement on rubbing the site of incision over the edge of the nest box when climbing it. Other, more traditional parameters of postoperative pain in animals, such as licking the incision site, droopiness, and obliviousness did not differ between the control and treatment group. Intuitively, the reaction in response to rubbing or touching the incision site indicating effectiveness of postoperative analgesic treatment makes sense. This parameter seems also to be a robust parameter in pain scales in dogs and cats.[18–20]

All the aforementioned behaviors are nonspecific and are also mentioned in descriptions of pain in other mammals. Pain-related behaviors in ferrets can, however, also be very subtle, as demonstrated in a study by Chattipakorn and colleagues.[7] This study established that the most significant behavioral change related to pain resulting from a tooth pulp inflammatory process was ipsilateral tongue protrusions, that is, the tongue protrusions were more often aimed toward the affected side. Other behaviors, such as face-wash strokes, headshakes, fore limb flails, paw-licks, ear grasps and chin rubs, seemed less specific. Most likely, such subtle behavioral changes are best detected by people spending a fair amount of time with the animal and observing it closely. In veterinary practice, these people are most likely to be the owner or veterinary technicians. It is therefore of pivotal importance to recognize the value of assessments made by the owner or technicians. The latter can be instructed to look for subtle changes in the animal's daily behavior. If frequent reports of specific behavioral signs are made in ferrets that are possibly in pain, these behaviors might be adopted for use in assessing pain in other individuals. To validate whether such behaviors are indeed related to pain, one can treat animals showing this behavior with analgesics, and evaluate the effect of the treatment on the display (attenuation or discontinuation) of the behavior. Although most of the signs of pain in ferrets currently reported seem relevant to acute postoperative pain, *home assessments* by the owner could also be valuable in detecting specific signs of chronic pain. In cats suffering from degenerative joint disease (DJD), for example, owners notice that the cats show a decrease in height and frequency of jumping, a reluctance to groom, and a decrease in food intake. Furthermore, these parameters seem strongly associated with radiological findings and are responsive to analgesic therapy.[21,22] In ferrets, the incidence of chronic pain due to, for example, DJD is unknown, and to date, the signs of chronic pain are not well documented. Similar to dogs and cats, one might expect ferrets with chronic pain to be hampered in their daily playful behavior, which might be easily noticed by the observant owner. However, such assessments are also prone to placebo effects, and therefore, should be interpreted with caution.[23,24]

Physiologic parameters, such as heart-rate and blood pressure, are sometimes used to assess pain in animals. However, because these parameters are not easily measured in ferrets and the restraint needed to record them would actually influence the recorded values, the mainstay of pain assessment in ferrets would be the behavioral assessment.[16]

Finally, many behavioral signs of pain in ferrets are described in the literature; however, the scientific evidence validating these parameters is limited. Effectiveness of analgesic therapy in ferrets can be assessed by observing and clinically examining the animal without costly equipment or complex procedures to make the assessment. All clinicians working with ferrets might develop their own pain scale for ferrets based on the experience of the clinic's employees for practical implementation in their specific clinic. Technicians and owners who spend a lot of time with the animals are invaluable in assessing the adequacy of analgesia, because they can quickly determine what is normal and abnormal for that individual animal. With minimal investment, a high gain can be achieved for adequate analgesic treatment and hence animal welfare.

PAIN PATHOPHYSIOLOGY

The basic approach to analgesic treatment in ferrets does not differ from the approach in humans and other commonly treated species, such as dogs and cats. Effective treatment of pain requires a basic understanding of the neuroanatomic and neuro-physiologic background of pain. This background is described in most handbooks about pain, anesthesia, and analgesia and is beyond the scope of this article.

Different classes of analgesic drugs can be used to stop or reduce the nociceptive input at different stages, that is, transduction, transmission, modulation, projection, and perception of the pain pathway. This is the basis of multimodal approach to pain management.[25] Transduction of pain can be influenced by local anesthetics and nonsteroidal anti-inflammatory drugs (NSAIDs); transmission, by local anesthetics, opioids, and alpha-2 agonists; modulation, by local anesthetics, NSAIDs, opioids, alpha-2 agonists, and N-Methyl D-Aspartate (NMDA) agonistic drugs; projection, by opioids, alpha-2 agonists, and NMDA agonistic drugs; and perception, by inhalational anesthetics, opioids, and alpha-2 agonists. The advantage of a multimodal approach is that different classes of analgesic drugs can have additive or synergistic effects. Furthermore, when using a combination of different analgesic drugs, the dose of the individual drugs can be lowered, which, in turn, might reduce side effects and increase safety.

Another important aspect of increasing the efficacy of analgesic therapy is preemptive analgesia. It has been shown in both humans and animals that previous experiences of pain can increase the aversiveness of subsequent painful events; although controversy on this topic persists,[26] pain might be treated best preemptively.

IMPLICATIONS OF THE UNIQUE PHYSIOLOGY OF FERRETS IN DESIGNING A PAIN MANAGEMENT PLAN

Diminished food and water intake in animals that are in pain can result in catabolic states and hypoglycemia in those with high metabolic rates.[10] Ferrets have short intestinal tracts and very fast intestinal transit times. Consequently, ferrets digest their food inefficiently.[27] The inefficient digestion and high metabolic rate of ferrets make them susceptible to developing a hypoglycemic state in the perianesthetic period.[28] The development of hypoglycemia can be enhanced by the presence of insulinoma (clinical or subclinical), which is common in companion ferrets.[29] Finally, inadequate pain treatment in ferrets recovering from surgery or suffering from critically illness might result in the development of hypoglycemia, which can potentially be life threatening. This underlines the pivotal importance of adequate monitoring and supportive care, including proper analgesic treatment, of ferrets.

Small animals, especially with long and thin bodies such as ferrets, are prone to develop hypothermia in the perianesthetic period. A field study anesthetizing free-ranging mink and polecats with ketamine and medetomidine reported a rapid decrease in body temperature after induction of anesthesia.[30] Inactivity due to inadequate pain treatment or overt sedation caused by analgesics can lead to the development of hypothermia, especially during postoperative recovery.[10] Because hypothermia is an important risk factor during the postoperative recovery period,[31] early intervention, including adequate analgesic support, and close monitoring in the postoperative period are of great importance in ferrets.

A study of the ferret liver's metabolizing of acetaminophen concluded that the activity of the hepatic enzyme glucuronosyltransferase in ferrets is similar to that in cats and that consequently, ferrets have a poor ability of glucuronidation of NSAIDs.[32] However, this was an in vitro study using microsomal preparations from frozen livers, and no in vivo results of the clearance of NSAIDs in ferrets were provided. Furthermore, it was concluded that ferrets do not share the same background that causes the relative poor activity of glucuronosyltransferase as cats. Also, glucuronidation is not the only way in which NSAIDs are metabolized or cleared from the body. Excretion of unchanged flunixin into the bile via organic anion transporters and thioesterification of ketoprofen are proposed as major excretion routes for these compounds in cats.[33] Therefore, in ferrets, other ways of metabolizing and excreting NSAIDs may also be present. Consequently, it cannot be readily concluded that ferrets have a diminished capacity for metabolizing and excreting NSAIDs similar to cats; however, it emphasizes the need for proper scientific studies into the pharmacodynamics and safety of NSAIDs and other analgesic drugs in ferrets. Until these studies are available, it might be prudent to extrapolate data on the use of NSAIDs in the cat to ferrets. Analogous with cats, close monitoring of the signs of side effects on the gastrointestinal tract and kidneys of the ferret is recommended when long-term use of NSAID is instituted.

THERAPEUTICS

As argued earlier, preemptive and multimodal analgesia, methodically intervening in the normal nociceptive pathway with different analgesics at the same and also distinct neuroanatomic levels, is part of effective pain management in humans and animals alike. The broad range of analgesic drugs used in more common companion species, such as dogs and cats, are also used in ferrets. Although the number of reports on analgesic efficacy, pharmacokinetics, and safety of the different drugs in ferrets is limited, a substantial number do exist on the clinical experience with these drugs. The reported doses, dose intervals, and routes of administration of the drugs described in the following sections are provided in **Table 1**.

NSAIDs

NSAIDs exert their effects by inhibiting the enzymes cyclo-oxygenase 1 and 2 (COX-1 and COX-2). The COX enzymes are responsible for the production of prostaglandins, among others, which play an important role in inflammatory processes and in regulating renal and gastrointestinal mucosal perfusion. The analgesic effects and the most important side effects, kidney failure and gastro-intestinal ulceration, are mediated by a reduction in the production of prostaglandins. A detailed description of the analgesic and side effects of NSAIDs goes beyond the scope of this article.

NSAIDs should be used with care for long-term treatment and are contraindicated in pregnant animals; animals with hepatic, renal, or gastrointestinal disorders; and/or animals that are in shock.[11] Contraindications for the use of NSAIDs are critically ill patients, preexisting renal disease, hypovolemia, bleeding disorders, and expected severe blood loss during surgery.[16] A recent report, however, states that preexisting renal disease is not necessarily a contraindication to the use of NSAIDs in cats,[34] but whether this also applies to ferrets is unclear currently. Pollock[35] states that NSAIDs are a poor choice for ferrets, because helicobacter gastritis and ulceration may develop with any concurrent stressor; however, there is no reference to support this statement. Based on the substantial number of reports on the successful use of NSAIDs in ferrets, these drugs can be considered a valuable additive to analgesic therapy in this species.

The use of meloxicam and carprofen, both potent COX-2 inhibitors, in ferrets is described by various authors.[16,35–38] Both drugs are stated to be relatively safe for ferrets and can be administered orally or by subcutaneous injection.[10,16,35] Flecknell[10] mentions that carprofen does not induce renal damage and therefore can be used

Table 1
Dose intervals and routes of administration of ferret analgesia drugs

Drug	Dose (mg/kg)	Route	Interval (h)	References
Opioids				
Buprenorphine	0.01–0.03	IV, IM, SC	8–12	10
	0.01–0.03	IM, PO, SC	6–10	11
	0.01–0.05	IV, SC	8–12	14
	0.01–0.03	IM, IV, SC	8–12	35
	0.004–0.01	IM, SC	6–8	39
Butorphanol	0.4	IM	4–6	10
	0.1–0.4	IM, IV, SC	2–4	11
	0.1–0.2 mg/kg/h CRI	IV		11
	0.1–0.5	IM, IV, SC	4–6	14
	0.1–0.2 loading dose followed by 0.1–0.2 mg/kg/h CRI	IV		16
	0.05–0.4	IM, SC	4–12	35
	0.2	IM, SC		39
Hydromorphone	0.1–0.2	IM, IV,SC	6–8	11
	0.05 loading dose followed by 0.05–0.1 mg/kg/h CRI	IV		16
Oxymorphone	0.05–0.2	IM, IV, SC	6–8	11
	0.05–0.2	IM, SC		35
Morphine	0.5–5	IM, SC	6	10
	0.05–0.5	IM, SC	2–6	35
Fentanyl	1–4 µg/kg/h CRI	IV		11
	2.5–5 µg/kg/h CRI (combined with ketamine CRI)	IV		16
Tramadol	10	PO	24	16
NSAIDS				
Meloxicam	0.1–0.2	PO, SC	24	11
	0.2 starting dose, followed by 0.1	IV, PO, SC	24	16
Carprofen	2.0–4.0	SC	24	10
	4.0	PO	24	16
	1.0–4.0	SC	12–24	35
Flunixin meglumine	0.5–2.0	SC	12–24	10
	1.1	PO, SC	14	14
	0.3–2.0	IV, PO, SC	24	35
Ketoprofen	1.0–2.0		24	16
	1.0–5.0	IM, PO	24	35
Other				
Ketamine	2.0 µg/kg/min	IV		11
	0.3–0.4 mg/kg/h with fentanyl CRI	IV		16
Medetomidine	0.001–0.002	IM,IV	4–6	16

Abbreviations: CRI, constant rate infusion; IM, intramuscular; IV, intravenous; PO, by mouth; SC, subcutaneous.

preoperatively, because no negative effects on renal function are expected when hypotension is encountered during surgery. However, the authors' do not know of any scientific data to support these statements.

Flunixin meglumine and ketoprofen, both potent COX-1 and COX-2 inhibitors, are described as being used in ferrets.[10,14,35] It is recommended that the latter drug is used with caution and only postoperatively, because of the expected negative effects on renal function and on the gastrointestinal mucosa.[10,16] However, no safety or toxicity studies for ferrets are available for either drug.

Finally, the authors consider NSAIDs valuable in analgesic therapy in the ferret. Since no clear safety studies are available, they should, however, be used with caution and/or appropriate monitoring intervals.

Opioids and Tramadol

Opioids exert their analgesic effects by agonistic effects on the opioid μ, κ, and/or δ receptor. The use of different types of opioids has been described in ferrets.

The use of buprenorphine in ferrets is described by various authors.[11,16,36–40] During a recent consensus meeting, buprenorphine was designated as a full μ-opioid receptor agonist in humans, with potent analgesic actions and few side effects, such as respiratory depression, nausea, and dysphoria.[41] Different authors assume different lengths for the duration of its analgesic actions, varying from 6 to 12 hours. It is reported that in ferrets, buprenorphine has profound sedative effects in the higher dose range.[11,14] Brown[14] suggests counteracting the sedative effects by giving naloxone at a dose of 0.04 mg/kg intravenously. However, antagonizing the sedative effects of opioids by the use of a full antagonist like naloxone also antagonizes the analgesic effects. In the human literature, there is controversy on this topic; however, several studies have demonstrated that naloxone can reverse the negative side effects of opioids, such as nausea, pruritus, and sedation, while keeping sufficient analgesia.[42,43] However, in animals, the lack of analgesia after (partially) antagonizing opioid effects by naloxone is not as readily assessable as in humans. Therefore, the authors advise to titrate opioids, especially those with a fast onset time (eg, morphine, methadone, fentanyl) to effect, but not to reverse the sedative effects with naloxone in ferrets. Furthermore, the authors advise that the animal be reassessed 30 to 60 minutes before the next dose of opioids, to identify inadequate long dose intervals or signs potentially associated with opioid adverse effects. When significant sedative effects or other negative side effects are encountered, the subsequent opioid dose can be reduced and the animal's analgesia reassessed.

Butorphanol is also frequently used to provide analgesia in ferrets.[11,14,16,36,39,44] It is assumed that butorphanol has agonistic effects on μ-, δ-, and κ-opioid receptors, with the highest affinity for the κ-opioid receptor.[45] Its clinical effects seem similar to buprenorphine; however, the duration of its analgesic actions seem significantly shorter—a maximum of 4 to 6 hours.[14,39] Therefore, the authors recommend the use of buprenorphine over butorphanol in ferrets.

The use of morphine, a μ-opioid receptor agonist,[46] in ferrets is reported.[10,11,35] Nausea and vomiting in response to morphine in its clinical dose range are described.[35] A study by Shiokawa and colleagues[47] also describes retching and vomiting in ferrets in response to the use of morphine in doses less than the clinical dose range—0.1, 0.3, and 0.6 mg/kg subcutaneously. Although this study used naïve, pain-free ferrets as an animal model to determine the antiemetic effect of aripiprazole, a partial dopamine D2 agonist, the findings support the clinical experience that morphine induces nausea and vomiting in the ferret. It might therefore be concluded that morphine should be used with caution in this species.

Methadone is a μ-opioid receptor agonist. In dogs, the incidence of methadone-associated vomiting was lower compared with morphine.[48] In humans, it is reported that opioid-associated side effects are lower when using methadone compared with morphine. However, strong scientific evidence to support this is lacking. Unlike in North America and the United Kingdom, methadone is readily available in mainland Europe. Therefore, it is used there more frequently than morphine in most species, except for the epidural and intra-articular route. In the authors' knowledge, the use of methadone in ferrets has not been described; however, it may be a valuable alternative to morphine in this species as well.

The use of hydromorphone and oxymorphone in ferrets, both μ-opioid receptor agonists,[46] is described.[11,16] For both agents, no clear descriptions exist of the clinical effects and duration thereof in ferrets. Based on the described dose intervals by Johnston,[11] clinical action can be assumed to last 6 to 8 hours.

The use of fentanyl, a short acting and very potent μ-opioid receptor agonist[46] with potent analgesic actions, has been described by Johnston[11] and Lichtenberger and Ko.[16] As in other species, fentanyl can be used as a constant rate infusion (CRI) in ferrets. Fentanyl CRI is most often used during surgery and in the postoperative period, but in the authors' opinion, can also be useful in trauma patients needing potent analgesia. Frequent reassessment, including ventilatory status and effectiveness of pain management, is mandatory in these patients.

The use of tramadol in the ferret has been described.[11,16] Tramadol is not a typical opioid. It is described to have effects on the μ-opioid receptor and the serotonin , the catecholamine, and the γ-aminobutyric acid systems. Tramadol is described as having significant analgesic effects in humans without inducing dependence.[46] In veterinary medicine, only a few studies on its analgesic effects in cats are available[49–51] and none, in dogs. The clinical effective dose in cats is 4 mg/kg with a dosing interval of 6 hours. This differs substantially from the dose and interval reported for the ferret by Lichtenberger and Ko,[16] that is, 10 mg/kg once daily. In cats, the palatability of tramadol is a significant clinical problem. Currently, its analgesic efficacy and palatability in ferrets is not described.

Finally, the clinical effects of opioids in ferrets seem to be similar to those in other species. Opioids, therefore, seem to be a valuable additive to analgesic therapy in ferrets. However, scientific evidence for the efficacy and pharmacokinetics in ferrets is generally lacking.

Alpha-2 Adrenoceptor Agonistic Drugs

The use of medetomidine, the alpha-2 adrenoceptor agonistic drug, has been recommended for ferrets in low doses, based on the presumed more profound cardiovascular depressant effects of the higher doses.[16] In dogs, low doses of medetomidine are indeed associated with fewer cardiovascular side effects[52]; however, these doses have limited sedative and/or analgesic effects. In the perioperative setting, alpha-2 adrenoceptor agonists have been shown to be well tolerated at sedative doses in cardiovascular-stable animals in a range of species. More recent human and veterinary literature indicates a place for the alpha-2 adrenoceptor agonists as part of pain management and/or sedation in an intensive-care setting as well.[53–57] Therefore, administration of alpha-2-agonistic drugs as low-dose CRI might also be a valuable additive to analgesic therapy and sedation in the ferret.

NMDA-Receptor Agonists

CRI of ketamine combined with CRI of fentanyl during and after surgery has been clinically described to provide good analgesia for the ferret.[16] Additionally, the use of ketamine CRI postoperatively has been recommended as an additive to analgesic therapy with opioids or other analgesics.[11]Although potentially very useful as analgesic adjuncts, ketamine and tiletamine, another NMDA-receptor agonist, are considered to have poor analgesic actions in the ferret[11,39] when used alone.

Local Anesthetics and Locoregional Techniques

Using local anesthetics, for example, bupivacaine and lidocaine, can be very effective in preventing stimuli reaching the spinal cord and are very useful additions in a pain management plan. The authors recommend that locoregional techniques are only performed in ferrets that are adequately sedated or anesthetized. The good predictability of drug effect with respect to desired and unwanted side effects of local anesthetics and insensitivity to species-specific physiology make locoregional techniques an excellent choice in ferrets requiring anesthesia for surgery or painful diagnostic procedures. Techniques that can be used in ferrets are incisional line blocks, local infiltration, ring blocks, splash blocks, topical application, conductive nerve blocks, and even epidural anesthesia.[10,11,16,35] Care must be taken not to exceed maximum doses, which need to be calculated beforehand, often requiring dilution of the drug to obtain an adequate volume. Maximum doses are similar to those for dogs and cats—1 to 2 mg/kg.[10,11,16] Adding opioids, such as morphine or buprenorphine, to a local block is considered to increase the duration of analgesia significantly.[16]

Specific dental blocks in ferrets are executed in a similar fashion to those in dogs and cats and were described in detail by Lichtenberger and Ko.[16] These included the infraorbital, mental, mandibular, and maxillary nerve blocks. Two other local blocks described by these investigators are the palatine and intratesticular blocks. In the latter, sufficient time has to be allowed for the local anesthetic to migrate to the spermatic cord (minimally, 5 minutes) to benefit from this technique.

The use of epidural morphine in the ferret at a dose of 0.1 mg/kg was reported to provide significant analgesia for 12 to 24 hours, with limited or no clinical side effects.[17] A 1:10 dilution of oxymorphone at 0.022 mg/kg for epidural analgesia has also been described.[35]

Finally, the locoregional techniques frequently used in dogs and cats should be actively pursued and their use encouraged in ferrets.

SUMMARY

A sufficient amount of data on clinical efficacy, pharmacokinetics, and pharmacodynamics of analgesic drugs and specific behaviors related to pain in ferrets is lacking. This might hamper effective pain management in both clinical and research settings. However, the authors think that ferrets do not differ from any other species when it comes to pain management. In pain management, the golden cycle is *assessment–intervention–reassessment.*

Assessment of pain is difficult in any species, including humans. Pain is a highly subjective and individual experience, and similar surgeries or disease states are experienced differently by every individual. Therefore, a patient-orientated pain management plan with strategic assessment intervals is strongly advocated, especially in species, such as the ferret, in which scientific data are scarce.

Finally, analgesic treatment is a dynamic, practical, and subjective process. Therefore, *clinical experience* from colleagues working with ferrets and with appropriate training in pain physiology and pain management is at least as valuable as *hard scientific* data. Therefore, the authors encourage people to maintain adequate record keeping and follow-up, while continuing to report on their clinical experience with anal-gesics in ferrets until more scientific evidence is available.

REFERENCES

1. Kehlet H, Holte K. Effect of postoperative analgesia on surgical outcome. Br J Anaesth 2001;87:62–72.
2. Bonnet F, Marret E. Postoperative pain management and outcome after surgery. Best Pract Res Clin Anaesthesiol 2007;21:99–107.
3. Cervero F. Afferent activity evoked by natural stimulation of the biliary system in the ferret. Pain 1982;13:137–51.
4. Bongenhielm U, Robinson PP. Afferent activity from myelinated inferior alveolar nerve fibers in ferrets after constriction or section and regeneration. Pain 1998; 74:123–32.
5. Long A, Bongenhielm U, Boissonade FM, et al. Neuropeptide immunoreactivity in ligature-induced neuromas of the inferior alveolar nerve in the ferret. Brain Res 1998;791:263–70.
6. Chattipakorn SC, Light AR, Willcockson HH, et al. The effect of fentanyl on c-fos expression in the trigeminal brainstem complex produced by pulpal heat stimu-lation in the ferret. Pain 1999;82:207–15.
7. Chattipakorn SC, Sigurdsson A, Light AR, et al. Trigeminal c-Fos expression and behavioral responses to pulpal inflammation in ferrets. Pain 2002;99:61–9.
8. Chattipakorn S, Chattipakorn N, Light AR, et al. Comparison of Fos expression within the ferret's spinal trigeminal nuclear complex evoked by electrical or noxious-thermal pulpal stimulation. J Pain 2005;6:569–80.
9. Loescher AR, Boissonade FM, Robinson PP. Calcitonin gene-related peptide modifies the ectopic discharge from damaged nerve fibres in the ferret. Neurosci Lett 2001;300:71–4.
10. Flecknell PA. Analgesia in small mammals. Semin Avian Exotic Pet Med 1998;7:41–7.
11. Johnston MS. Clinical approaches to analgesia in ferrets and rabbits. Semin Avian Exotic Pet Med 2005;14:229–35.
12. Jha SK, Coleman T, Frank MG. Sleep and sleep regulation in the ferret (Mustela putorius furo). Behav Brain Res 2006;172:106–13.
13. Thurber A, Jha SK, Coleman T, et al. A preliminary study of sleep ontogenesis in the ferret (Mustela putorius furo). Behav Brain Res 2008;189:41–51.
14. Brown SA. Clinical techniques in domestic ferrets. Semin Avian Exotic Pet Med 1997;6:75–85.
15. Pollock C. Emergency medicine of the ferret. Vet Clin North Am Exot Anim Pract 2007;10:463–500.
16. Lichtenberger M, Ko J. Anesthesia and analgesia for small mammals and birds. Vet Clin North Am Exot Anim Pract 2007;10:293–315.
17. Sladky KK, Horne WA, Goodrowe KL, et al. Evaluation of epidural morphine for postoperative analgesia in ferrets (Mustela putorius furo). Contemp Top Lab Anim Sci 2000;39:33–8.
18. Hardie EM, Hansen BD, Carroll GS. Behavior after ovariohysterectomy in the dog: what's normal? Appl Anim Behav Sci 1997;51:111–28.
19. Firth AM, Haldane SL. Development of a scale to evaluate postoperative pain in dogs. J Am Vet Med Assoc 1999;214:651–9.
20. Murrell JC, Psatha EP, Scott EM, et al. Application of a modified form of the Glas-gow pain scale in a veterinary teaching centre in the Netherlands. Vet Rec 2008; 162:403–8.

21. Bennett D, Morton C. A study of owner observed behavioural and lifestyle changes in cats with musculoskeletal disease before and after analgesic therapy. J Feline Med Surg 2009;11:997–1004.

22. Slingerland LI, Hazewinkel HA, Meij BP, et al. Cross-sectional study of the prevalence and clinical features of osteoarthritis in 100 cats. Vet J 2010. [Epub ahead of print].

23. Lascelles BD, Court MH, Hardie EM, et al. Nonsteroidal anti-inflammatory drugs in cats: a review. Vet Anaesth Analg 2007;34:228–50.

24. Brown DC, Boston RC, Coyne JC, et al. Ability of the canine brief pain inventory to detect response to treatment in dogs with osteoarthritis. J Am Vet Med Assoc 2008;233:1278–83.

25. Kehlet H, Dahl JB. The value of "multimodal" or "balanced analgesia" in postoperative pain treatment. Anesth Analg 1993;77:1048–56.

26. Dahl JB, Møiniche S. Pre-emptive analgesia. Br Med Bull 2004;71:13–27.

27. Bell JA. Ferret nutrition. Vet Clin North Am Exot Anim Pract 1999;2:169–92.

28. Ko J, Marini RP. Anesthesia and analgesia in ferrets. In: Fish RE, Brown MJ, Danneman PJ, et al, editors. Anesthesia and analgesia in laboratory animals. San Diego (CA): Elsevier; 2008. p. 443–56.

29. Chen S. Pancreatic endocrinopathies in ferrets. Vet Clin North Am Exot Anim Pract 2008;11:107–23.

30. Fournier-Chambrillon C, Chusseau JP, Dupuch J, et al. Immobilization of free-ranging European mink (Mustela lutreola) an polecat (Mustela putorius) with medetomidine-ketamine and reversal by atipamezole. J Wildl Dis 2003;39:393–9.

31. Burger L, Fitzpatrick J. Prevention of inadvertent perioperative hypothermia. Br J Nurs 2009;18:1114, 1116–9.

32. Court MH. Acetaminophen UDP-glucuronosyltransferase in ferrets: species and gender differences, and sequence analysis of ferret UGT1A6. J Vet Pharmacol Ther 2001;24:415–22.

33. Lascelles BD, Hansen BD, Roe S, et al. Evaluation of client-specific outcome measures and activity monitoring to measure pain relief in cats with osteoarthritis. J Vet Intern Med 2007;21:410–6.

34. Sparkes AH, Heiene R, Lascelles BD, et al. ISFM and AAFP consensus guidelines: long-term use of NSAIDs in cats. J Feline Med Surg 2010;12:521–38.

35. Pollock C. Postoperative management of the exotic animal patient. Vet Clin North Am Exot Anim Pract 2002;5:183–212.

36. Darby C, Ntavlourou V. Hepatic hemangiosarcoma in two ferrets (Mustela putorius furo). Vet Clin North Am Exot Anim Pract 2006;9:689–94.

37. Jekl V, Hauptman K, Jeklová E, et al. Hydrometra in a ferret-case report. Vet Clin North Am Exot Anim Pract 2006;9:695–700.

38. Vinke CM, van Deijk R, Houx BB, et al. The effects of surgical and chemical castration on intermale aggression, sexual behaviour and play behaviour in the male ferret (Mustela putorius furo). Appl Anim Behav Sci 2008;115:104–21.

39. Evans TA, Springsteen KK. Anesthesia of ferrets. Semin Avian Exotic Pet Med 1998;7:48–52.

40. Hermann BA, Plensdorf KL, Degner DA. Medical and surgical management of traumatic elbow luxation in a juvenile ferret. Vet Clin North Am Exot Anim Pract 2006;9:651–5.

41. Pergolizzi J, Aloisi AM, Dahan A, et al. Current knowledge of buprenorphine and its unique pharmacological profile. Pain Pract 2010. [Epub ahead of print].

42. Gan TJ, Ginsberg B, Glass PS, et al. Opioid-sparing effects of a low-dose infusion of naloxone in patient-administered morphine sulfate. Anesthesiology 1997;87:1075–81.

43. Maxwell LG, Kaufmann SC, Bitzer S, et al. The effects of a small-dose naloxone infusion on opioid-induced side effects and analgesia in children and adolescents treated with intravenous patient-controlled analgesia: a double-blind, prospective, randomized, controlled study. Anesth Analg 2005;100:953–8.
44. Morera N, Valls X, Mascort J. Intervertebral disk prolapse in a ferret. Vet Clin North Am Exot Anim Pract 2006;9:667–71.
45. Commiskey S, Fan LW, Ho IK, et al. Butorphanol: effects of a prototypical agonist-antagonist analgesic on kappa-opioid receptors. J Pharmacol Sci 2005;98: 109–16.
46. Trescot AM, Datta S, Lee M, et al. Opioid pharmacology. Pain Physician 2008;11: S133–53.
47. Shiokawa M, Narita M, Nakamura A, et al. Usefulness of the dopamine system-stabilizer aripiprazole for reducing morphine-induced emesis. Eur J Pharmacol 2007;570:108–10.
48. Monteiro ER, Junior AR, Assis HM, et al. Comparative study on the sedative effects of morphine, methadone, butorphanol or tramadol, in combination with acepromazine, in dogs. Vet Anaesth Analg 2009;36:25–33.
49. Brondani JT, Loureiro Luna SP, Beier SL, et al. Analgesic efficacy of perioperative use of vedaprofen, tramadol or their combination in cats undergoing ovariohysterectomy. J Feline Med Surg 2009;11:420–9.
50. Castro DS, Silva MF, Shih AC, et al. Comparison between the analgesic effects of morphine and tramadol delivered epidurally in cats receiving a standardized noxious stimulation. J Feline Med Surg 2009;11:948–53.
51. Pypendop BH, Siao KT, Ilkiw JE. Effects of tramadol hydrochloride on the thermal threshold in cats. Am J Vet Res 2009;70:1465–70.
52. Pypendop BH, Verstegen JP. Hemodynamic effects of medetomidine in the dog: a dose titration study. Vet Surg 1998;27:612–22.
53. Lin GY, Robben JH, Murrell JC, et al. Dexmedetomidine constant rate infusion for 24 hours during and after propofol or isoflurane anaesthesia in dogs. Vet Anaesth Analg 2008;35:141–53.
54. Riker RR, Shehabi Y, Bokesch PM, et al. Dexmedetomidine vs midazolam for sedation of critically ill patients: a randomized trial. JAMA 2009;301:489–99.
55. Valtolina C, Robben JH, Uilenreef J, et al. Clinical evaluation of the efficacy and safety of a constant rate infusion of dexmedetomidine for postoperative pain management in dogs. Vet Anaesth Analg 2009;36:369–83.
56. Shehabi Y, Nakae H, Hammond N. The effect of dexmedetomidine on agitation during weaning of mechanical ventilation in critically ill patients. Anaesth Intensive Care 2010;38:82–90.
57. Tan JA, Ho KM. Use of dexmedetomidine as a sedative and analgesic agent in critically ill adult patients: a meta-analysis. Intensive Care Med 2010;36:926–39.

Tramadol Use in Zoologic Medicine

Marcy J. Souza, DVM, MPH, DABVP (Avian), DACVPM*,
Sherry K. Cox, MS, PhD

KEYWORDS

- Tramadol • Analgesia • Opioid receptors • Zoologic medicine
- Exotic animal medicine

THE NEED FOR ANALGESIA IN ZOOLOGIC SPECIES

Analgesia is becoming increasingly important in veterinary medicine, and controlling pain in zoologic animals is an important component to improving the welfare of captive animals. Behaviors associated with pain are variable between species, and some animals may not show signs until severely distressed. Careful observation of behavior by animal care staff can aid in the recognition and therefore treatment of painful conditions in zoologic animals.

Numerous analgesics are available for use in animals, but a few have been extensively used or studied in zoologic species. Tramadol is a new analgesic that is available in an inexpensive oral form and is not controlled. Tramadol may be an alternative to other analgesics, such as opioids and nonsteroidal antiinflammatory drugs, when treating acute or chronic pain in zoologic animals.

MECHANISM OF ACTION OF TRAMADOL

Tramadol is a centrally acting analgesic drug that is licensed and used in humans.[1] Its analgesic efficacy is a result of complex interactions between the opiate, adrenergic, and serotonin receptor systems.[1] It is both a weak opioid agonist with selectivity for the μ-receptor (opioid μ receptor) and a weak inhibitor of the reuptake of norepinephrine and serotonin (5-hydroxytryptamine). This dual mechanism of action may be attributed to the 2 enantiomers of racemic tramadol. The 2 enantiomers act synergistically to provide analgesia. The S(+) enantiomer of tramadol has a low affinity for μ-receptors. This enantiomer inhibits the cellular reuptake of serotonin and increases its extracellular release. The R(−) enantiomer more effectively inhibits norepinephrine reuptake and increases its cellular release by autoreceptor activation.[1,2] Tramadol provides analgesia mainly via the serotonin and norepinephrine pathways.

Department of Comparative Medicine, College of Veterinary Medicine, University of Tennessee, 2407 River Drive, Knoxville, TN 37996, USA
* Corresponding author.
E-mail address: msouza@utk.edu

Vet Clin Exot Anim 14 (2011) 117–130
doi:10.1016/j.cvex.2010.09.005
1094-9194/11/$ – see front matter © 2011 Elsevier Inc. All rights reserved.
vetexotic.theclinics.com

Hepatic demethylation of tramadol produces the active metabolite O-desmethyltramadol (M1), which also exists as a racemic mixture. The S(+)-M1 interacts with μ-receptors, whereas R(−)-M1 interacts with α_2-adrenergic receptors.[3] The S(+)-M1 is reported to be 2 to 200 times more potent in μ-receptor binding as S(+)-tramadol.[4,5] A large portion of the analgesic effect of tramadol is because of the M1 metabolite[6–8]; thus, a variability in the biotransformation of tramadol into M1 might clearly affect the analgesic effect and treatment response.

The demethylation reaction to produce M1 in humans is metabolized by the cytochrome P450 (CYP) 2D6 isoenzyme (CYP2D6).[9,10] CYP2B6 and CYP3A4 are also primarily involved in the formation of metabolites, M5 and M3, respectively.[11,12] The wide variability in the pharmacokinetic properties of tramadol in human beings can partly be attributed to CYP genetic polymorphism.[9] The existence of different alleles in humans results in functionally different enzymes.[13] Studies in humans also indicate that biphasic kinetics occur for the formation of the metabolites M1 and M2, which indicates the participation of more than one CYP isoform in the tramadol metabolism pathway.[13] Because of the large degree of variation in metabolism, pharmacokinetic parameters must be established for each species. The pharmacokinetics of tramadol and its metabolites have been reported in humans,[1,13] dogs,[14–18] cats,[19–21] horses,[22–26] goats,[27] donkeys,[28] llamas,[29] and camels.[30] Several studies indicate interspecies differences in drug metabolism.

Opioid peptides of the mammalian central nervous system are grouped into 3 families: the enkephalin, the dynorphin, and the endorphin peptides. These peptide families exert their effects on the nervous system by interacting with 3 specific endogenous opiate receptors.[31] Opioid peptides have been found in the nervous system of all classes of vertebrates, including amphibians, reptiles, and birds, and many different invertebrate groups.[31] Opioid drugs mediate their effects by binding to G protein–coupled receptors that are also activated by endogenously produced opioid neuropeptides. The 3 pharmacologically distinct types of mammalian opioid receptors μ, δ, and κ are encoded by separate structural genes.[32] μ-Receptors are of primary importance for mediating the effects of opioid drugs in mammals and play a role in other vertebrates as well. These receptors are present in the brains of birds,[31] reptiles,[33] amphibians,[34] and fish.[35] The distribution of μ-receptors depends on the species as well as on the region of the brain examined. Opioid κ and δ receptors (κ- and δ-receptors, respectively) are also present across species, and studies in birds have suggested that κ-receptors may be more important than μ-receptors in producing analgesia.[36]

Tramadol has a wide margin of safety in humans, with minimal respiratory, cardiovascular, or gastrointestinal side effects.[1,13,37] Opioid analgesics are generally associated with respiratory depression, which is mediated through a decrease in the sensitivity of the respiratory center to carbon dioxide that results in a decrease in the respiratory rate. Studies in humans indicate that unlike other opioids, tramadol is not likely to produce clinically significant respiratory depression.[1] Tramadol has no clinically relevant effects on blood pressure or heart rate. In healthy human patients, heart rate and blood pressure were only slightly elevated after intravenous (IV) administration of tramadol.[13] In contrast to other μ-receptor agonists, tramadol has only minor effects on gastric emptying. In a long-term study, tramadol was found to have only a minor delay on colonic transit time but no effect on upper gastrointestinal tract transit or gut smooth muscle tone.[13]

Tramadol and M1 also inhibit the reuptake of norepinephrine (noradrenaline) and serotonin, which are important activating components of the descending pain inhibitory system.[37–39] When the descending pain inhibitory system is activated, the transmission of painful stimuli through the dorsal horn of the spinal cord is inhibited by the action of endogenous opioids.[39] By inhibiting the reuptake of both norepinephrine and serotonin, tramadol activates the descending pain inhibitory system, therefore decreasing the sensation of pain. These 2 mechanisms of action of tramadol, binding to opioid receptors and activation of the descending pain inhibitory system, work synergistically to provide analgesia in vertebrate species. One study also suggested that tramadol may provide analgesia by antagonizing N-methyl-D-aspartate (NMDA) receptors.[40] NMDA receptors are located throughout the nervous system, as well as in the viscera. Antagonism of NMDA receptors reduces the hyperexcitability of nociceptive neurons in the dorsal horn of the spinal cord, therefore decreasing pain.[41,42] Other metabolites, including M2, M3, M4, and M5, have been described, but it is unknown whether they have analgesic properties.[7]

Tramadol can interact with selective serotonin reuptake inhibitors and monoamine oxidase inhibitors, so tramadol should be used with caution in patients on these medications.[1] Also, concomitant administration of carbamazepine, cimetidine, and quinidine results in their interaction with tramadol, and hence, they should be used cautiously.[1] Patients with opiate sensitivity could experience dysphoria, agitation, and sedation as possible side effects to administration of tramadol.

At present, only oral preparations of tramadol are available in the United States; however, injectable preparations are available in Europe and South America. Unlike morphine and other opioids, tramadol is not a scheduled drug controlled by the Drug Enforcement Agency, a component of the US Department of Justice.

TRAMADOL USE IN HUMANS AND DOMESTIC ANIMALS
Humans

Tramadol is rapidly absorbed after a single or multiple oral doses of 100 mg in adult volunteers.[1] The elimination half-life after a single oral (100 mg) or parenteral (50 mg) dose in adults was 5.5 hours, whereas the half-life of M1 after oral doses was 6.69 hours.[1] Grond and Sablotzki[13] reviewed multiple human studies and found that the half-life of tramadol ranged from 5 to 6 hours. Tramadol half-life is roughly increased by 2-fold in patients with renal or hepatic impairment. M1 is the primary metabolite formed in humans; however, there are interindividual differences in metabolism, which may be due to the genetic polymorphism of CYP2D6.[43] The most common side effects in humans are nausea, dizziness, drowsiness, tiredness, sweating, and vomiting.

The analgesic efficacy of IV, intramuscular (IM) and oral tramadol has been established in extensive studies in adult patients with moderate to severe acute postoperative pain.[1,13] Tramadol has also been used in the treatment of posttraumatic, obstetric, and renal pain. Parenteral or oral tramadol was effective in relieving moderate to severe postoperative pain associated with several types of surgery, by reducing pain intensity by 47% to 58% within 4 to 6 hours.[1] The overall analgesic efficacy of tramadol is comparable to that achieved using equianalgesic doses of parenteral morphine or alfentanil.

In humans, the reported minimally effective analgesic plasma concentrations range from 298 ± 171 ng/mL to 590 ± 410 ng/mL for tramadol and 39.6 ± 29.5 ng/mL to 84 ± 34 ng/mL for M1.[44,45] It has been suggested that in humans, the clinically effective target plasma concentration of tramadol to treat mild to moderate pain can be as low as 100 ng/mL.[46]

Dogs

The use of tramadol in dogs has been investigated in several studies.[14–18] The pharmacokinetics of tramadol and its active metabolite M1 was determined after IV and oral administration of tramadol at 4.4 mg/kg and 100 mg, respectively, to 6 adult beagles.[14]

No adverse effects were noted after either dose; however, dogs administered with 1 mg/kg of M1 exhibited signs of nausea, including salivation and increased swallowing. After IV and oral administration, the half-life of tramadol was 1.80 and 1.71 hours, whereas the half-life of M1 was 1.69 and 2.18 hours, respectively. The maximum concentration (C_{max}) for tramadol after oral administration was 1402.75 ng/mL, whereas that of M1 after IV and oral administration was 146.90 and 449.13 ng/mL, respectively. Kukanich and Papich[14] suggest that the short elimination half-life of M1 after oral tramadol administration to dogs would require frequent dosing to maintain target plasma concentrations but steady state would be reached rapidly. They also suggest that M1 is a minor metabolite in dogs when compared with other metabolites not measured. Based on the information from their study a simulated oral dosing regimen of 5 mg/kg every 6 hours or 2.5 mg/kg every 4 hours is predicted to produce tramadol and M1 concentrations that are consistent with producing analgesia in humans. McMillan and colleagues[15] also found that M1 was present but at very low levels after 1, 2, and 4 mg/kg of IV administration to 6 male mixed breed dogs. The low levels of M1 detected and the close proximity to the lower limit of quantification, which was between 9.8 and 1937 ng/mL, did not permit the evaluation of pharmacokinetic parameters. One dog in the study developed nausea and increased salivation after each dose, and sedation scores increased with increasing doses in all dogs. There were no effects on heart or respiratory rates after any of the doses. McMillan and colleagues[15] also suggest that the rapid elimination rate has implications when designing dosage regimens in dogs and may result in failure of analgesia if canine dosage regimens are based on human studies. Dogs require more frequent doses to maintain adequate therapeutic drug concentrations.

Vettorato and colleagues[16] found that M1 was a prominent metabolite after IV administration of 2 mg/kg of tramadol to dogs for surgery. Variable concentrations of both tramadol (5.00–0.09 µg/mL) and M1 (0.35–0.09 µg/mL) were noted in the study. Breeds, gender, body weight, and ages were not standardized, and it is suggested that these factors might have influenced the variable M1 formation rate. Tramadol was administered extradurally to dogs undergoing tibial plateau leveling osteotomy and found to produce adequate intra- and postoperative analgesia without significant side effects. However, the analgesia produced was not superior to that obtained after IV administration; therefore, the extradural route was considered an impractical alternative to IV tramadol administration in dogs.

Giorgi and colleagues[17,18] examined the profile of tramadol in dogs in 2 different studies. In the first study, 100 mg of tramadol was given IV, IM, orally (immediate and sustained release capsules), and rectally to 6 male beagles.[17] After IV and IM injections, animals exhibited some side effects such as excitation and tremors but these effects were transient and resolved within 1 hour. In the second study, 4 mg/kg of tramadol was administered via suppositories and IV injection to 6 male beagles.[18] There were no adverse effects after either dose. The half-life for tramadol was 1.02 and 2.24 hours after IV and rectal administration, respectively, whereas the C_{max} after rectal administration was 134 ng/mL. M1 was detected in negligible amounts near the limit of quantification, which was 5 ng/mL.

Based on a descriptive and visual analog scale, Mastronique and Fantoni[47] found that in 30 female dogs of different breeds and ages undergoing ovariohysterectomy, the analgesic effects of IV tramadol (2.0 mg/kg) were equivalent to those produced by IV morphine (0.2 mg/kg). In a recent study on electroencephalographic responses to acute noxious electric stimulation responses, tramadol, parecoxib, and morphine were compared in anaesthetized dogs.[48] The study found that morphine (0.5 mg/kg subcutaneously) prevented any increase in F50 (median frequency) after noxious electric stimulation, whereas both tramadol (3.0 mg/kg subcutaneously) and pare-coxib failed to prevent an increase in F50 because of uninhibited nociceptive transmission to the cerebral cortex in response to the same stimuli.

Seddighi and colleagues[49] studied the effects of tramadol on the minimum alveolar concentration (MAC) of sevoflurane in dogs. They found that tramadol significantly reduced the MAC, but it was not dose dependent at the doses studied, which ranged from 1.5 to 3.0 mg/kg.

Cats

Pypendop and Ilkiw[19] administered 2 mg/kg IV and 5 mg/kg oral tramadol to 6 adult female cats. No adverse effect was observed after either dose; in fact, the cats appeared euphoric for several hours. After IV and oral administration, the half-life of tramadol was 2.23 and 3.40 hours, whereas the half-life of M1 was 4.35 and 4.82 hours, respectively. The C_{max} for tramadol was 1323 and 914 ng/mL, whereas that of M1 was 366 and 655 ng/mL after IV and oral administration, respectively. This result is similar to the results obtained in another study in which tramadol was administered at 2 mg/kg IV and had a half-life of 2.18 hours.[20] Pypendop and Ilkiw[19] suggest M1 is one of the main metabolites produced in cats. Pypendop and colleagues[21] continued their work in cats with a study on the pharmacodynamic effects of tramadol. Oral doses of 0.5, 1.0, 2.0, and 4.0 mg/kg tramadol in gelatin capsules were used, which produced mean plasma tramadol levels from 25.8 to 539.8 ng/mL and mean M1 levels from 94.5 to 480.4 ng/mL. They found that tramadol did induce thermal antinociception in cats; however, doses of 2 mg/kg or more were necessary to yield a significant and sustained effect. This result agrees with results from another study in which tramadol administered at 1 mg/kg subcutaneously had minimal or no effect on thermal and mechanical thresholds in cats.[50] Some of the behavioral and physical effects, such as euphoria and mydriasis, observed after administration of tramadol were similar to the classic effects observed after administration of moderate doses of opioids in cats. No clinically important adverse effects were observed in the cats for any of the doses. Data from the study suggested that to achieve 95% of the maximum thermal antinociceptive effect of tramadol, plasma concentrations of approximately 350 ng/mL would have been required. This concentration would be within the range of higher concentrations that provide postoperative analgesia in humans. Simulation based on pharmacokinetic parameters for tramadol in cats reported in another study and pharmacodyanmics of this study by Pypendop and Ilkiw[19] predict that administration of 4 mg/kg tramadol every 6 hours results in plasma tramadol concentrations of 350 ng/mL or more for 89% of the time overall and more than 90% of the time after the last 3 doses.

Ko and colleagues[51] studied the effects of tramadol on the MAC of sevoflurane in cats. Results indicated that oral administration of tramadol reduced MAC of sevoflurane and that the magnitude of this effect was an intermediate between that of butorphanol and hydromorphone. This reduction was thought to be because of tramadol's effects on opioid receptors and was reversible with the administration of naloxone. Analgesic effects of tramadol were also compared with those of morphine after their epidural administration in cats, and tramadol was found to provide analgesia for the first 6 hours after administration.[52]

Goats

DeSousa and colleagues[27] examined the pharmacokinetics of tramadol after an oral and IV administration of 2 mg/kg tramadol to 6 female goats. No adverse effects were noted after either dose. The half-life for tramadol was 0.94 and 2.67 hours after IV and oral administration, respectively. Tramadol levels were measurable for 3 and

2 hours after oral and IV administration, respectively, with a C_{max} of 542.9 ng/mL after the oral dose and an initial concentration (C_0) of 3200.0 ng/mL after the IV dose.

M1 was in detectable levels after IV administration and had a half-life of 2.89 hours but was not detectable in the plasma after the oral dose. Based on information from the study it was suggested that an IV dose of 4 mg/kg given every 6 hours should produce tramadol and M1 concentrations consistent with analgesia in humans. To date, no pharmacodynamic studies have been done with tramadol in goats to evaluate the analgesic efficacy.

Camels

One study has determined the pharmacokinetics of tramadol in camels. Elghazali and colleagues[30] administered 2.33 mg/kg of tramadol via IV and IM injections to 6 (3 male, 3 female) healthy camels. No adverse effects were observed after either dose. The half-life of tramadol was 1.3 and 3.2 hours after IV and IM administration, respectively. The C_{max} and C_0 of tramadol were 0.44 and 1.40 μg/mL after IV and IM dosing, respectively. M1 was detected in urine but was not quantified. As yet, no pharmacodynamic studies have been done with tramadol in this species to evaluate the analgesic effectiveness.

Llamas

In a study, 6 adult male llamas were administered 2 mg/kg tramadol either IV or IM[29] Adverse effects were observed during the IV administration in the last llama, which had muscle twitching and ataxia. This effect lasted for roughly 15 minutes, after which no further adverse effects were observed; however, no adverse effects were noted after IM administration. The half-life for tramadol was 2.12 and 2.54 hours, whereas the half-life for M1 was 10.40 and 7.73 hours after IV and IM administration, respectively. After IV and IM administration, tramadol concentrations ranged from 4036 to 9 ng/mL and 1360 to 9 ng/mL, whereas M1 concentrations ranged from 158 to 39 ng/mL and 158 to 29 ng/mL, respectively. Based on information from the study, a simulated oral dosing regimen of 4 mg/kg of tramadol given IM every 12 hours is predicted to lead to plasma concentrations in the average animal, which are associated with analgesia in humans. To date, no pharmacodynamic studies have been conducted with tramadol in this species to evaluate the analgesic effectiveness.

Donkeys

In a study conducted by Giorgi and colleagues,[28] 12 male donkeys received a dose of 2.5 mg/kg tramadol either IV or orally (immediate release capsule). Tramadol half-life was 1.5 and 4.2 hours after IV and oral administration, respectively, and no adverse effects were observed with either dose. The C_{max} for tramadol after oral administration was 2817 ng/mL. After IV administration, M1 concentrations were higher than the minimum effective plasma concentration of 80 ± 60 ng/mL reported in humans, for a period of 5 minutes to 8 hours, which suggested a long-acting effectiveness of the drug. There was a limited production of M1 after oral administration, which may result in decreased analgesic efficacy when this route is used. To date, no pharmaco-dynamic studies have been performed with tramadol in this species to evaluate the analgesic effectiveness. Clinical effectiveness of tramadol has been questioned in species that mainly metabolize it to inactive metabolites, suggesting that this drug may not be an effective and safe analgesic in humans.

Horses

There are several studies involving the use of tramadol in horses.[22–26] Tramadol was administered IV to 5 horses (male and female) at a dose of 2.5 mg/kg in a study conducted by Zonca and colleagues.[25] No adverse effects were observed in the treated animals. The half-life of tramadol was 1.29 hours, and although M1 was present in quantifiable concentrations in all samples, no further information was provided. These results are similar to those seen in another study in which 5 horses were administered tramadol, 2 mg/kg IV, and the half-life was 1.36 hours.[22] However, adverse effects were observed during IV administration in the first 2 animals, which had muscle twitching that lasted 10 to 15 minutes. These effects occurred when tramadol was administered over 5 to 6 minutes. When tramadol administration was prolonged to 10 minutes, the adverse effects were not observed. Shilo and colleagues[22] administered tramadol IM and orally to 7 horses, and the half-life and C_{max} of tramadol were 1.53 hours and 637 ng/mL, respectively, after IM administration; however, absorption was poor after oral administration, with only 3% found in systemic circulation, and therefore half-life was not calculated. The C_{max} of tramadol after the oral dose was 33 ng/mL. Very low levels of M1 were also detected after IV, IM and oral administration.[22] Similar adverse effects were observed in a study in which horses were administered tramadol (2 mg/kg) IV, and hence, this portion of the study was discontinued.[26] However, tramadol was administered orally (2 mg/kg) to the same horses, with no adverse effects. The half-life for tramadol and M1 was 10.10 and 4.00 hours, respectively. The concentrations in this study ranged from 256 to 15 ng/mL and 47 to 11 ng/mL for tramadol and M1, respectively.

Giorgi and colleagues[23] administered tramadol, 5 mg/kg, IV to horses, and similar to other studies, the animals exhibited adverse effects, such as nausea, confusion, agitation, tremors, and tachycardia, in varying degrees. The effects started within 3 to 5 minutes of administration and resolved 2 hours after dosing. The plasma concentrations of M1 in this study[23] were only marginal, in agreement with the results of Shilo and colleagues.[22]

Dhanjal and colleagues[24] conducted a study on both the pharmacokinetics and pharmacodynamics of tramadol, 2 mg/kg, after its administration to 7 horses. Some side effects were evident, such as head nodding, sensitivity to noise, excitation, increased alertness, and trembling, which occurred in 5 of the 6 horses. The half-life and C_{max} for tramadol after IV administration were 2.05 hours and 2.2 μg/mL, respectively, and M1 concentrations were not quantified in the study. Tramadol, however, did not produce analgesia in the horses as determined by their response to a thermal nociceptive stimulus.

TRAMADOL USE IN ZOOLOGIC SPECIES

A few studies examining tramadol in zoologic species have been published; some are reviewed in the following sections. Research is available for several species regarding the efficacy of opioids, particularly morphine and other μ opioids; however, literature concerning the role of norepinephrine and serotonin in the analgesia of zoologic species is scant. Because of the lack of published studies or clinical trials using tramadol, dosing in zoologic species must often be estimated based on clinician experience or extrapolation from pharmacokinetic and pharmacodynamic studies in other species. Studies performed in domestic animals, as reviewed previously, can be tremendously helpful when choosing a dose of tramadol for a particular zoologic species. In addition, plasma concentrations of tramadol and M1 associated with analgesia have not been reported for zoologic species, with the exception of recent studies in parrots.[53]

Delivering medication to zoologic animals can be a challenge. Tramadol is commercially available as 50-mg tablets that can be hidden in food items that are eaten whole, such as meatballs, small rodents, and fish. Some animals may be unwilling to take the medication in a pill form, and a compounded suspension of tramadol has been evaluated for stability.[54] Wagner and colleagues[54] mixed crushed tramadol tablets with 1 of the 2 commercial suspension agents and found that both the solutions maintained approximately 99% of the initial drug concentration after 90 days at room temperature. Flavors can also be added to these suspensions to make them more palatable for various species.

Fish and Amphibians

One study found that analgesia was achieved when carps (*Cyprinus carpio*) were administered tramadol before an electric thermal stimulus.[55] Analgesia was dose dependent, lasted for 2 hours, and did not affect swimming or normal behaviors when compared with controls. Other studies have provided evidence that fish have similar nociceptive processing systems and opioid receptors as terrestrial mammals.[35,56,57] Studies are needed to determine the metabolism and analgesic efficacy of tramadol in various fish species.

Studies have been conducted to examine the opioid affinity and function of μ-receptors in frogs.[34] One study found that slight and profound analgesia was obtained after giving low-dose (10 mg/kg) and high-dose (100 mg/kg) morphine, respectively, in frogs (*Rana pipiens pipiens*) with no noticeable behavioral effects.[58] No reports of tramadol use in clinical cases or research in amphibians have been published, but μ-receptors are present and may play a role in analgesia.

Reptiles

Greenacre and colleagues[59] examined the analgesic effect of tramadol in bearded dragons (*Pogona vitticeps*) after a noxious electric stimulus. There was significant analgesia after oral administration of tramadol, 11 mg/kg. Another study showed that high-dose morphine (10 and 20 mg/kg) had analgesic effects in bearded dragons after a noxious thermal stimulus.[60] These studies suggest that μ-receptors may be primarily responsible in opioid-induced analgesia in bearded dragons. Further studies are needed to examine tramadol in other species of lizards to determine appropriate dosing regimens.

Research in turtles has suggested that opioid-mediated analgesia is primarily associated with μ-receptor activation, with a small contribution from δ-receptor activation.[61] Respiratory depression after μ- and δ-receptor activation has been reported in turtles.[62] A recent study found that when red-eared sliders were orally dosed with tramadol at 10 mg/kg, they had a delayed withdrawal from a noxious thermal stimulus when compared with controls.[63] This analgesic effect was present for 6 to 96 hours after dosing. Similar effects were observed with subcutaneous dosing but for a shorter duration postdosing (12–48 hours). The investigators concluded that when red-eared sliders were dosed orally with tramadol at 10 mg/kg, long-lasting effective analgesia was achieved.

No studies examining tramadol in snakes have been published. Response to opioids seems to be variable between species of snakes. One study examined physiologic responses (plasma cortisol and catecholamine levels, blood pressure, heart rate) of ball pythons (*Python regius*) after surgery and found no difference in control animals versus animals dosed with either meloxicam (0.3 mg/kg) or butorphanol (5.0 mg/kg).[64] The investigators concluded that at the doses administered, neither meloxicam nor butorphanol seemed to provide postoperative analgesia to ball pythons. Another study found that high doses of butorphanol (20 mg/kg), but not morphine, induced analgesia after a noxious thermal stimulus in corn snakes (*Elaphe guttata*).[60] Species-specific research may be required with snakes to determine the role of various opioid receptors and the analgesia-associated doses of tramadol.

A few studies addressing analgesia have been performed in crocodilians. One study evaluated the efficacy of morphine in crocodiles (*Crocodylus niloticus africana*) after a noxious thermal stimulus.[65] Morphine was injected intraperitoneally and doses of 0.5 to 1.0 mg/kg were found to provide antinociceptive effects. No research examining tramadol use in crocodilians is available.

Birds

Numerous studies have examined analgesics in several avian species. A pharmacodynamic study in African gray parrots (*Psittacus erithacus*) found that κ-agonists, such as butorphanol, were more effective analgesics than μ-agonists, such as buprenorphine.[36] One study in chickens found that administration of both μ- and κ-agonists led to a reduction of isoflurane minimum anesthetic concentration.[66] Fentanyl, a μ-agonist, administered to white cockatoos (*Cacatua alba*) produced analgesia, but some birds became hyperactive after administration.[67] A review of published avian analgesic studies shows a wide range of responses to administration of μ- and κ-opioids, indicating that both μ- and κ-receptors may play a role in opioid-mediated analgesia.

Tramadol has been examined in several avian species including bald eagles (*Haliaetus leucocephalus*),[68] red-tailed hawks (*Buteo jamaicensis*),[7,69] peafowl (*Pavo cristatus*),[70] and Hispaniolan Amazon parrots (*Amazon ventralis*).[53] Pharmacokinetic parameters varied between species.

The studies in bald eagles and red-tailed hawks did not involve the evaluation of tramadol's analgesic efficacy; the objective in both studies was to report the pharmacokinetics of a single dose of tramadol.[68,69] Recommended doses for raptors ranged from 5 mg/kg twice a day (bald eagles) to 8 mg/kg twice a day (red-tailed hawks). These doses were based on plasma concentrations of tramadol in eagles and hawks, which were in the same range as analgesic concentrations in humans. Clinically, with the above-mentioned dosages raptors become sedated after numerous doses; therefore, less-frequent administration or lower doses may be required for repeat dosing. Further studies in raptors examining pharmacodynamics, as well as the pharmacokinetics of repeat dosing, are needed.

Six peafowl were administered oral tramadol, and blood was collected over time.[70] Initial findings indicated that less-frequent dosing, possibly only once daily, would likely be needed to maintain plasma concentrations that are associated with analgesia in humans. Similar to raptors, further studies would be beneficial to examine species differences in metabolism and efficacy of the drug.

The pharmacodynamics and pharmacokinetics of tramadol are currently being evaluated in Hispaniolan Amazon parrots.[53] Initial data suggest that oral doses of 30 mg/kg are required to provide analgesia in response to a noxious thermal stimulus. This dose of tramadol provided significant analgesia for 6 hours after dosing when compared with controls. This higher dose may be necessary because of differences in absorption and metabolism when compared with other birds. Additional studies examining tramadol in Amazon parrots are being conducted at present. The initial findings in Amazon parrots reemphasize the importance of species-specific pharmacokinetic and pharmacodynamic research not only for birds but also for zoologic species in general.

Mammals

Tramadol use in various mammalian zoologic species has been reported,[71–73] but research has only been performed in a few species, predominately rodents and rabbits. Dosing is typically extrapolated from published studies in other closely related mammalian species.

A few studies have been performed in rodents, primarily in a laboratory animal medicine setting. One study found that intraperitoneally administered tramadol (10 mg/kg) abolished postoperative hyperalgesia in rats when compared with saline or parecoxib.[74] Another study in a rat experimental model suggested that oral tramadol doses as low as 0.45 mg/kg may provide analgesia; the researchers also found that tramadol can provide localized analgesia when administered subcutaneously at the site that would receive a noxious stimulus.[75] The same study suggested that tramadol and gabapentin may work synergistically to provide analgesia for rats. Rats administered with varying doses of intraperitoneal tramadol (1–25 mg/kg) showed delayed responses after thermal or ischemic noxious stimuli but they may have decreased motor function at higher doses.[76] In a clinical setting, tramadol is most commonly administered orally, and unfortunately, currently available research has not used this route of administration. Rodent studies examining the analgesic pharmacodynamics of tramadol at various oral doses are needed.

Rabbits were administered oral tramadol at 11 mg/kg, and blood samples were collected at various time points up to 6 hours postdosing.[77] Although the plasma tramadol and M1 concentrations associated with analgesia in rabbits are not known, these concentrations were less than those associated with analgesia in humans. The investigators concluded that administering oral tramadol at 11 mg/kg is unlikely to provide analgesia to rabbits for a clinically acceptable length of time. The low plasma tramadol concentrations in rabbits are similar to those found after oral dosing in horses. Another study evaluated the effect of tramadol on MAC of isoflurane (ISOMAC) in rabbits.[78] After IV administration of tramadol (4.4 mg/kg), there was a significant reduction of ISOMAC, but this reduction was thought to be clinically unimportant. Plasma tramadol and M1 concentrations at the time of ISOMAC reduction ranged from 181 to 636 ng/mL and 32 to 61 ng/mL, respectively. Until further research is conducted to determine appropriate oral doses, tramadol should be paired with another mode of analgesia, such as a nonsteroidal antiinflammatory drug, when used in rabbits.

SUMMARY

Tramadol may be an alternative to analgesics currently used in zoologic medicine. A few studies examining the effect of tramadol in zoologic species are available and they suggest that significant species differences exist in pharmacokinetics as well as analgesic dynamics. Until more research is available, recommended doses will be based solely on clinical experience. Clinicians at various zoologic institutions and exotic clinical practices are encouraged to perform clinical trials and aid in the determination of appropriate doses of tramadol for the many zoologic species present.

REFERENCES

1. Scott LJ, Perry CM. Tramadol: a review of its use in perioperative pain. Drugs 2000;60:139–76.
2. Raffa RB, Friderichs E, Reimann W, et al. Opioid and nonopioid components independently contribute to the mechanism of action of tramadol, an atypical opioid analgesic. J Pharmacol Exp Ther 1992;280:275–85.
3. Valle M, Garrido MJ, Pavon JM, et al. Pharmacokinetic-pharmacodynamic modeling of the antinociceptive effects of main active metabolites of (-)-O-des-methyltramadol, in rats. J Pharmacol Exp Ther 2000;293:646–53.

4. Hennies HH, Friderichs E, Schneider J. Receptor binding, analgesic and antitussive potency of tramadol and other selected opioids. Arzneimittelforschung 1988; 38:877–80.

5. Poulsen L, Arendt-Nielsen L, Brosen K, et al. The hypoanalgesic effect of tramadol in relation to CYP2D6. Clin Pharmacol Ther 1996;60:636–44.

6. Gillen C, Haurand M, Kobelt D, et al. Affinity, potency and efficacy of tramadol and its metabolites at the cloned human mu-opioid receptor. Naunyn Schmiedebergs Arch Pharmacol 2000;362:116–21.

7. Wu W, McKown L, Gauthier A, et al. Metabolism of the analgesic drug, tramadol hydrochloride, in rat and dog. Xenobiotica 2001;31:423–41.

8. Parker R. Tramadol. Compend Contin Educ Pract Vet 2004;26:800–2.

9. Abdel-Rahman S, Leeder J, Wilson J. Concordance between tramadol and dextromethorphan parent/metabolite ratios: the influence of CYP2D6 and non-CYP2D6 pathways on biotransformation. J Clin Pharmacol 2002;42:24–9.

10. Pedersen R, Damkier P, Brosen K. Enantioselective pharmacokinetics of tramadol in CYP2D6 extensive and poor metabolizers. Eur J Clin Pharmacol 2006;62: 513–21.

11. Chen H, Chen W, Gan L, et al. Metabolism of (S)-5, 6-Difluoro-4-cyclopropyle-thynyl-4-trifluoromethyl-3, 4-dihydro-2(1H)-quinazolinone, a non-nucleoside reverse transcriptase inhibitor, in human liver microsomes. Metabolic activation and enzyme kinetics. Drug Metab Dispos 2003;31:122–32.

12. Subrahmanyam V, Renwick A, Walters D, et al. Identification of cytochrome P-450 isoforms responsible for cis-tramadol metabolism in human liver microsomes. Drug Metab Dispos 2001;29:1146–55.

13. Grond S, Sablotzki A. Clinical pharmacology of tramadol. Clin Pharm 2004;43: 779–923.

14. Kukanich B, Papich MG. Pharmacokinetics of tramadol and the metabolite O-desmethyltramadol in dogs. Vet Pharmacol Ther 2004;27:239–46.

15. McMillan CJ, Livingston A, Clark CR, et al. Pharmacokinetics of intravenous tramadol in dogs. Can J Vet Res 2008;72:325–31.

16. Vettorato E, Zonca A, Isola M. Pharmacokinetics and efficacy of intravenous and extradural tramadol in dogs. Vet J 2009. [Epub ahead of print]. DOI: 10.1016/j.tvjl.2008.11.002.

17. Giorgi M, Del Carlo S, Saccomanni G, et al. Biopharmaceutical profile of tramadol in the dog. Vet Res Commun 2009;33(Suppl 1):S189–92.

18. Giorgi M, Del Carlo S, Saccomanni G, et al. Pharmacokinetics of tramadol and its major metabolites following rectal and intravenous administration in dogs. N Z Vet J 2009;57:146–52.

19. Pypendop BH, Ilkiw JE. Pharmacokinetics of tramadol and its metabolite O-desmethyl-tramadol, in cats. Vet Pharmacol Ther 2007;31:52–9.

20. Cagnardi P, Zonca A, Carli S, et al. Pharmacokinetics of tramadol in cats undergoing neutering. J Vet Pharmacol Ther 2006;29(Suppl 1):289–90.

21. Pypendop BH, Siao KT, Ilkiw JE. Effects of tramadol hydrochloride on the thermal threshold in cats. Am J Vet Res 2009;70:1465–70.

22. Shilo Y, Britzi M, Eytan B, et al. Pharmacokinetics of tramadol in horses after intravenous, intramuscular and oral administration. J Vet Pharmacol Ther 2007;31: 60–5.

23. Giorgi M, Soldani G, Manera C, et al. Pharmacokinetics of tramadol and its metabolites M1, M2 and M5 in horses following intravenous, immediate release (fasted/fed) and sustained release single dose administration. J Equine Vet Sci 2007;27:481–8.

24. Dhanjal JK, Wilson DV, Robinson E, et al. Intravenous tramadol: effects, nociceptive properties, and pharmacokinetics in horses. Vet Anaesth Analg 2009;36:581–90.
25. Zonca A, Cagnardi P, Carli S, et al. Pharmacokinetics of tramadol in horses. J Vet Pharmacol Ther 2006;29(Suppl 1):290–1.
26. Cox S, Villarino N, Doherty T. Determination of oral tramadol pharmacokinetics in horses. Res Vet Sci 2010;89:236–41.
27. DeSousa AB, Santos AC, Schramm SG, et al. Pharmacokinetics of tramadol and o-desmethyltramadol in goats after intravenous and oral administration. Vet Pharmacol Ther 2007;31:45–51.
28. Giorgi M, Del Carlo S, Sgorbini M, et al. Pharmacokinetics of tramadol and its metabolites M1, M2, and M5 in donkeys after intravenous and oral immediate release single-dose administration. J Equine Vet Sci 2009c;29:569–74.
29. Cox S, Martin-Jimenez T, Doherty T. Pharmacokinetics of intravenous and intramuscular tramadol in llamas. J Vet Pharmacol Ther, 2010. [Epub ahead of Print]. DOI: 10.1111/j.1365-2885.2010.01219.x.
30. Elghazali M, Barezaik IM, Abdel Hadi AA, et al. The pharmacokinetics, metabolism and urinary detection time of tramadol in camels. Vet J 2008;178:272–7.
31. Reiner A, Brauth SE, Kitt CA, et al. Distribution of mu, delta, and kappa opiate receptor types in the forebrain and midbrain of pigeons. J Comp Neurol 1989;280:359–82.
32. Von Zastrow M, Svingos A, Haberstock-Debic H, et al. Regulated endocytosis of opioid receptors: cellular mechanisms and proposed roles in physiological adaptation to opiate drugs. Curr Opin Neurobiol 2003;13:348–53.
33. Xia Y, Haddad GG. Major difference in the expression of delta- and mu-opioid receptors between turtle and rat brain. J Comp Neurol 2001;436:202–10.
34. Brassel CM, Sawyer GW, Stevens CW. A pharmacological comparison of the cloned frog and human mu opioid receptors reveals differences in opioid affinity and function. Eur J Pharmacol 2008;599:36–43.
35. Neiffer DL, Stamper MA. Fish sedation, analgesia, anesthesia, and euthanasia: considerations, methods, and types of drugs. ILAR J 2009;50:343–60.
36. Paul-Murphy JR, Brunson DB, Miletic V. Analgesic effects of butorphanol and buprenorphine in conscious African grey parrots (Psittacus erithacus erithacus and Psittacus erithacus timneh). Am J Vet Res 1999;60:1218–21.
37. Leppert W, Luczak J. The role of tramadol in cancer pain treatment - a review. Support Care Cancer 2005;13:5–17.
38. Tramadol [package insert]. Detroit (MI): Caraco Pharmaceutical Laboratories Ltd; 2006.
39. Yoshimura M, Furue H. Mechanisms for the anti-nociceptive actions of the descending noradrenergic and serotonergic systems in the spinal cord. J Pharm Sci 2006;101:107–17.
40. Hara K, Minami K, Sata T. The effects of tramadol and its metabolite on glycine, gamma-aminobutyric acid, and N-methyl-D-aspartate receptors expressed in Xenopus oocytes. Anesth Analg 2005;100:1400–5.
41. Pozzi A, Muir WW, Traverso F. Prevention of central sensitization and pain by N-methyl-D-aspartate receptor antagonists. J Am Vet Med Assoc 2006;228:53–60.
42. Petrenko AB, Yamakura T, Baba H, et al. The role of N-methyl-D-aspartate (NMDA) receptors in pain: a review. Anesth Analg 2003;97:1108–16.
43. Gan SH, Ismail R, Wan Adnan WA, et al. Impact of CYP2D6 genetic polymorphism on tramadol pharmacokinetics and pharmacodynamics. Mol Diagn Ther 2007;11:171–81.
44. Grond S, Meuser T, Uragg H. Serum concentrations of tramadol enantiomers during patient-controlled analgesia. Br J Clin Pharmacol 1999;48:254–7.

45. Lehmann K, Kratzenberg U, Schroeder-Bark B, et al. Postoperative patient-controlled analgesia with tramadol: analgesic efficacy and minimum effective concentrations. Clin J Pain 1990;6:212–20.
46. Malone H, Sonet B, Streel B, et al. Pharmacokinetic evaluation of a new oral sustained release dosage form of tramadol. Br J Clin Pharmacol 2004;57:270–8.
47. Mastronique S, Fantoni DT. A comparison of preoperative tramadol and morphine for the control of early postoperative pain in canine ovariohysterectomy. Vet Anaesth Analg 2003;30:220–8.
48. Kangara K, Chambers JP, Johnson CB. Electroencephalographic responses of tramadol, parecoxib and morphine to acute noxious electrical stimulation in anaesthetized dogs. Res Vet Sci 2010;88:127–33.
49. Seddighi MR, Egger CM, Rohrbach B, et al. Effects of tramadol on the minimum alveolar concentration of sevoflurane in dogs. Vet Anaesth Analg 2009;36:334–40.
50. Steagall PVM, Taylor PM, Brondani JT, et al. Antinociceptive effects of tramadol and acepromazine in cats. J Feline Med Surg 2008;10:24–31.
51. Ko JC, Abbo LA, Weil AB, et al. Effect of orally administered tramadol alone or with an intravenously administered opioid on minimum alveolar concentration of sevoflurane in cats. J Am Vet Med Assoc 2008;232(12):1834–40.
52. Castro DS, Silva MFA, Shih AC, et al. Comparison between the analgesic effects of morphine and tramadol delivered epidurally in cats receiving a standardized noxious stimulation. J Feline Med Surg 2009;11:948–53.
53. Souza MJ, Guzman DS, Paul-Murphy J, et al. Tramadol in Hispaniolan Amazon parrots (*Amazona ventralis*). In: Proceedings of Association of Avian Veterinarians. San Diego (CA); 2010. p. 293–4.
54. Wagner DS, Johnson CE, Cichon-Hensley BK, et al. Stability of oral liquid preparations of tramadol in strawberry syrup and a sugar-free vehicle. Am J Health Syst Pharm 2003;60:1268–70.
55. Chervova LS, Lapshin DN. Opioid modulation of pain threshold in fish. Dokl Biol Sci 2000;375:590–1.
56. Braitwaithe VA, Boulcott P. Pain perception, aversion and fear in fish. Dis Aquat Org 2007;75:131–8.
57. Newby NC, Robinson JW, Vachon P, et al. Pharmacokinetics of morphine and its metabolites in freshwater rainbow trout (*Oncorhynchus mykiss*). J Vet Pharmacol Ther 2008;31:117–27.
58. Pezalla PD. Morphine-induced analgesia and explosive motor behavior in an amphibian. Brain Res 1983;273:297–305.
59. Greenacre CB, Massi K, Schumacher JP, et al. Comparative antinociception of various opioids and non-steroidal anti-inflammatory medications versus saline in the bearded dragon (*Pagona vitticeps*) using electrostimulation. In: Proceedings of the Association of Reptilian and Amphibian Veterinarians. Los Angeles (CA); 2008. p. 87.
60. Sladky KK, Kinney ME, Johnson SM. Analgesic efficacy of butorphanol and morphine in bearded dragons and corn snakes. J Am Vet Med Assoc 2008;233:267–73.
61. Sladky KK, Kinney ME, Johnson SM. Effects of opioid receptor activation on thermal antinociception in red-eared slider turtles (*Trachemys scripta*). Am J Vet Res 2009;70:1072–8.
62. Johnson SM, Kinney ME, Wiegel LM. Inhibitory and excitatory effects of micro-, delta-, and kappa-opioid receptor activation on breathing in awake turtles, *Trachemys scripta*. Am J Physiol Regul Integr Comp Physiol 2008;295:R1599–612.

63. Cummings BB, Sladky KK, Johnson SM. Tramadol analgesic and respiratory effects in red-eared slider turtles (*Trachemys scripta*). In: Proceedings of American Association of Zoological Veterinarians and American Association of Wildlife Veterinarians Joint Conference. Tulsa (OK); 2009. p. 115.

64. Olesen MG, Bertelsen MF, Perry SF, et al. Effects of preoperative administration of butorphanol or meloxicam on physiologic responses to surgery in ball pythons. J Am Vet Med Assoc 2008;233:1883–8.

65. Kanui TI, Hole K. Morphine and pethidine antinociception in the crocodile. J Vet Pharmacol Ther 1992;15:101–3.

66. Concannon KT, Dodam JR, Hellyer PW. Influence of mu- and kappa-opioid agonist on isoflurane minimal anesthetic concentration in chickens. Am J Vet Res 1995;56:806–11.

67. Hoppes S, Flammer K, Hoersch K, et al. Disposition and analgesic effects of fentanyl in white cockatoos (*Cacatua alba*). J Avian Med Surg 2003;17:124–30.

68. Souza MJ, Martin-Jimenez T, Jones MP, et al. Pharmacokinetics of oral and intravenous tramadol in bald eagles. J Avian Med Surg 2009;23:247–52.

69. Souza MJ, Martin-Jimenez T, Jones MP, et al. Pharmacokinetics of oral tramadol in red tailed hawks, J Vet Pharm Therap, 2010. [Epub ahead of Print]. DOI: 10.1111/j.1365-2885.2010.01211.x.

70. Black PA, Cox S, Macek M, et al. Pharmacokinetics of tramadol hydrochloride and its metabolite O-desmethyltramadol in peafowl (*Pavi crustatys*). In: Proceedings of American Association of Zoological Veterinarians and American Association of Wildlife Veterinarians Joint Conference. Tulsa (OK); 2009. p. 109.

71. Ramsay EC. Use of analgesics in exotic felids. In: Fowler ME, Miller RE, editors, Zoo and wild animal medicine, current therapy, vol. 6. St Louis (MO): Saunders Elsevier; 2008. p. 289–93.

72. Spriggs M, Arble J, Myers G. Intervertebral disc extrusion and spinal decompression in a binturong (*Arctictis binturong*). J Zoo Wildl Med 2007;38:135–8.

73. McCain S, Souza MJ, Schumacher JP, et al. Surgical correction of occipital bone proliferation associated with hypovitaminosis A in a lion. J Zoo Wildl Med 2007; 39:421–7.

74. Kamermann P, Koller A, Loram L. Postoperative administration of the analgesic tramadol, but not the selective cyclooxygenase-2 inhibitor parecoxib, abolishes postoperative hyperalgesia in a new model of postoperative pain in rats. Pharmacology 2007;80:244–8.

75. Granados-Sato V, Arguelles CF. Synergic antinociceptive interaction between tramadol and gabapentin after local, spinal and systemic administration. Pharmacology 2005;74:200–8.

76. Loran LC, Mitchell D, Skosana M, et al. Tramadol is more effective than morphine and amitriptyline against ischaemic pain but not thermal pain in rats. Pharm Res 2007;56:80–5.

77. Souza MJ, Greenacre CB, Cox SK. Pharmacokinetics of oral tramadol in the domestic rabbit. Am J Vet Res 2008;69:979–82.

78. Egger CM, Souza MJ, Greenacre CB, et al. Isoflurane sparing effects of intravenous tramadol in the domestic rabbit. Am J Vet Res 2009;70:945–9.

Zoologic Companion Animal Rehabilitation and Physical Medicine

Jessica K. Rychel, DVM[a],*, Matthew S. Johnston, VMD, DABVP (Avian)[b],
Narda G. Robinson, DO, DVM, MS[a]

KEYWORDS

• Exotics • Zoologic animals • Rehabilitation • Pain management
• Massage • Therapeutic laser

Similar to traditional pet species, zoologic companion animals are subject to illness and injury. Therefore it is important to recognize not only the merits of traditional analgesia for these species but also the benefits of physical medicine. Physical medicine is an all-encompassing term that refers to the use of mechanical touch and physical modalities including cryotherapy, heat therapy, laser therapy, massage, and rehabilitation. Physical medicine can be an integral part of recovery from trauma and surgery for veterinary patients and typically has fewer adverse effects than conventional medicine, yet it can aid in a more rapid and complete recovery. Zoologic companion animals sometimes struggle with conventional medical interventions and may recover more slowly than other species, making these patients natural candidates for rehabilitation.

PAIN EVALUATION AND ANALGESIA: AN ESSENTIAL FIRST STEP

Regardless of the species presented, the ability to assess pain in an individual patient is essential before beginning any form of physical medicine. A discussion of pain recognition and traditional pharmacologic analgesia in zoologic companion animals is beyond the scope of this article, but the reader is referred to previous work on this subject.[1] Ethical considerations and performance ability should be taken into account when working with patients with managed or poorly managed pain. Patients with pain cannot perform therapeutic exercise as effectively, and rehabilitation becomes

The authors have nothing to disclose.
[a] Department of Clinical Sciences, Center for Comparative and Integrative Pain Medicine, Colorado State University, 300 West Drake Road, Fort Collins, CO, 80523, USA
[b] Department of Clinical Sciences, Colorado State University, 300 West Drake Road, Fort Collins, CO, 80523, USA
* Corresponding author.
E-mail address: jessicarychel@gmail.com

unpleasant for the patient, client, and veterinarian if the exercises make the patient uncomfortable. Although rehabilitation and physical medicine can provide some analgesia, in cases in which severe pain is present these modalities need to be augmented by additional treatments including local pain control measures, pharmaceutical intervention, acupuncture, and related techniques. Appropriate analgesia for a wide variety of zoologic companion animals is discussed in other articles in this issue.

CRYOTHERAPY

Cryotherapy, the application of cold therapy to an injured area, is often used to reduce pain and inflammation during the acute phase of injury. Cold packs applied to an acute injury reduce pain by slowing nociceptor transmission from the area. Cryotherapy also reduces pain by causing vasoconstriction, which lessens local edema and inflammation, and slows the release of histamines and other inflammatory mediators at the site of injury by limiting blood flow and local cellular metabolism, further offsetting pain and uncomfortable postoperative swelling.[2] Cryotherapy provides effective analgesia at little cost, and owners can be taught to apply this therapy for their companion animal at home, as long as they receive appropriate information about the risks and safe application. Rabbits and ferrets recovering from surgery are excellent candidates for routine basic cryotherapy as shown in **Fig. 1**. Ice packs are rolled into a light towel and applied to the surgical incision at 10- to 15-minute intervals 3 to 4 times daily in the first 1 to 2 days after operation. Subjectively, the authors have observed a decrease in incisional complications, such as swelling and self-mutilation, since instituting this therapy.

Small exotic companion animals can chill easily, therefore, the body temperature needs to be monitored and accounted for when considering the use of cold therapy for an injury. For example, cryotherapy may be contraindicated in the immediate postoperative period or just after an injury because the patient may be hypothermic. It is also important to monitor patients carefully while applying ice packs to ensure that they are not having an adverse topical reaction and that their core body temperature remains stable. Cryotherapy may cause deleterious local or systemic effects in reptiles, amphibians, and fishes because the ectothermic physiology of these species precludes safe use. Chilling ectothermic animals reduces immune function, which is essential for recovery from injury and illness.[3–5]

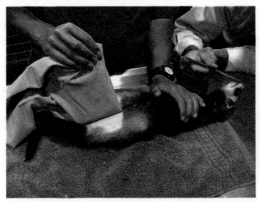

Fig. 1. A ferret with a postoperative abdominal incision receives cryotherapy while eating a treat.

THERAPEUTIC LASER

Therapeutic laser is recommended for wound healing and analgesia, and this technique continues to gain application in veterinary medicine, including for zoologic companion species (**Fig. 2**). This technique has few risks and contraindications and is often beneficial. Although the complete mechanism of action of therapeutic laser is not well understood, when applied to an injured region it seems to improve circulation,[6] encourage normalized neurologic function,[7,8] affect local and regional inflammation,[6,9,10] and ease pain in the injured area.[11,12] It has also been shown that therapeutic laser can improve collagen deposition[13] and collagen density in injury healing, which improves superficial wound healing, hastens bone healing, and speeds the recovery period after an orthopedic injury.[14] Patients with a reduced bone density caused by nutritional secondary hyperparathyroidism or other causes recover faster when treatment is supplemented with laser therapy. Although this condition is common to certain companion reptiles, these models have not been studied specifically.[15] Published studies of laser therapy for zoologic companion animals are few, although one case report involving laser therapy as part of a multimodal approach to neuropathic pain management in a prairie falcon demonstrates that laser therapy may assist in pain reduction and wound healing.[16]

Therapeutic laser can be safely applied to most species, although the safety and penetration of laser through the thick epidermis of reptiles and fishes is unknown. In all species, laser is contraindicated during pregnancy and in juvenile animals with

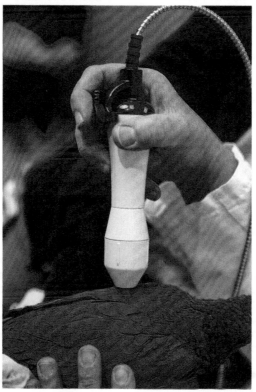

Fig. 2. Therapeutic laser is beneficial for a wide variety of conditions, including wound healing, pain management, and orthopedic and neurologic injuries.

open growth plates because its heating effect could prematurely close growth plates or have other adverse effects. Laser therapy should be avoided in patients with cancer, particularly at the tumor site, because it could potentiate cell growth. Laser should also be used with caution in small patients because it can quickly accumulate superficial heat, which may be painful or cause a burn. Patients' eyes should always be protected from direct laser light to avoid retinal damage. The optimal dose of laser has not yet been determined, although 1 to 5 J/cm^2 provides an effective treatment in most cases. Laser doses up to 60 J/cm^2 have been reported to be beneficial.[8,10,11]

THERAPEUTIC EXERCISE

Therapeutic exercise encompasses a wide variety of activities, which can be creative and enjoyable for patients and pet owners. A few key principles should be kept in mind when prescribing therapeutic exercise for zoologic companion animals. The most important aspect of therapeutic exercise is to avoid pain or further injury, and the recommended exercises should be natural and enjoyable for the patient to perform. If therapeutic exercise becomes a struggle for the patient, it is unreasonable to continue forcing the patient to perform these tasks. The goals for therapeutic exercise include strengthening, improving or maintaining range of motion of the joints and spine, and building proprioception and stability.[17]

Beginning with basic movement and assisted standing after an orthopedic or a neurologic injury is important. Assisting patients first into sternal recumbency and then to standing helps them build strength and balance to stand on their own, which leads to greater independence, the ability to eat and drink on their own, improved circulation, better lung function,[18–20] and a more effective transition to advanced therapeutic exercise. Good footing is important in the early stages of rehabilitation while the patient's balance and strength are being restored. Helping patients to relearn standing can be difficult if they are skittish, so devices such as slings or harnesses may be used. In addition, supportive devices such as carts can be made. There are companies that design carts for rabbits and other small mammals.

Performing passive range of motion exercises is an effective means of keeping joints moving appropriately as a patient recovers from injury, but it is essential that these exercises are done with extreme caution, particularly in small fragile patients that are susceptible to subsequent injury even with gentle handling. If owners will be performing passive range of motion exercises at home, they should be educated to look for signs of pain or discomfort. These exercises should be used to maintain current range of motion, not to push or stretch so hard that a soft tissue tear or fracture could occur. Passive range of motion exercise is considered an essential postoperative therapy after an orthopedic repair of most wing injuries; without exercise the propatagial tendon can become irreversibly contracted.[21–23]

As patients regain strength and coordination they can progress to more active therapeutic exercise, improvised according to the patient's species, specific goals, and abilities. Avian examples include weight shifting on a balance board, perching on a perch that is slightly movable, walking up and down an incline, and walking on an uneven or unsteady surface. Specific exercises can also be designed to strengthen specific muscle groups, such as lifting a small weight, step-up exercises, or maneuvering around an obstacle.

HEAT THERAPY

Warming an injured area is not appropriate in the acute inflammatory phase, but patients with chronic pain or old injuries may find superficial heat from a hot pack soothing and enjoyable. Superficial heat therapy reduces pain by reducing sympathetic neurologic tone, promoting circulation, and reducing muscle spasms. Heat therapy applied across the abdominal wall can also improve gastrointestinal motility,[24] likely because of the reduction in sympathetic tone and reduced pain sensation. Finally, heat therapy can speed healing because of its ability to increase tissue oxygenation, improve local circulation, and speed biochemical reactions. However, such therapy can also cause increased tissue destruction in the cases in which abundant degradative enzymes are present.[2]

Hot packs should be applied with caution and are contraindicated in patients with fever, acute inflammatory pain or difficulty with thermoregulation. If a patient reacts negatively to heat therapy, the treatment should be discontinued because the patient may experience increased pain as a result of heat. Extreme caution should be exercised when using hot pack therapy in sedated and anesthetized patients or those with decreased sensation caused by their disease process. Many zoologic companion species have delicate skin that burns more easily than that of cats and dogs, so in these species it is best to use hot packs only if the patient has normal sensation and an ability to move away from the heat source.

Therapeutic ultrasound is another modality used for heat application, but in this case the heat penetrates more deeply and is sometimes better tolerated than heat packs.[25] Therapeutic ultrasound can be used for heating muscles with contracture, particularly problematic in avian species after orthopedic wing repairs or prolonged wing bandaging. Treatment with therapeutic ultrasound can reduce contracture and improve range of motion in the affected joints when applied several times weekly[26] during bandage changes, before passive range of motion exercise or therapeutic exercise, and after a cast or bandage is removed in the final stages of healing and rehabilitation.

MASSAGE THERAPY

Massage therapy can be beneficial in many species for pain relief, anxiety reduction, and promotion of the human-animal bond. For these reasons, massage that is appropriately done can be rewarding for pet owners and pleasant for patients (**Fig. 3**). Gentle massage can help reduce edema, improve pain, and reduce sympathetic tone.

Gentle massage attuned to the patient's needs and tolerance can be applied by nursing staff and pet owners with proper training. Massaging the abdominal wall has been shown to improve postoperative ileus in humans,[27] and by extrapolation

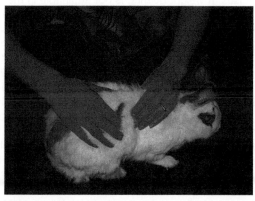

Fig. 3. A geriatric rabbit receiving massage therapy to reduce discomfort associated with widespread osteoarthritis.

and based on the authors' experience, is beneficial in small companion mammals such as rabbits, chinchillas, and guinea pigs. Putative mechanisms of massage performed with moderate pressure involve stimulation of vagal afferent fibers in the viscera as well as the abdominal wall.[28] Heightened vagal activity increases and/or regulates gastric motility as demonstrated in preterm human infants.[29,30]

Massage therapy for musculoskeletal ailments in humans improves range of motion,[31] dissipates myofascial restriction, treats pain, reduces anxiety, and elevates mood.[32,33] Given these positive effects and the safety of conscientiously performed massage, soft tissue manual therapy techniques such as massage play a prominent role in caring for rabbits and other small mammals experiencing myofascial and mechanical dysfunctions associated with head tilt.

SPECIFIC INJURIES
Orthopedic Injuries

Small mammals, birds, and reptiles are prone to orthopedic injuries, particularly fractures, because of their small size and thin cortices. Fractures and orthopedic injuries of all kinds are universally painful for animals and can be life threatening because of shock, pain, and secondary dysfunction, such as ileus. To minimize pain and secondary illness, rehabilitation modalities should be used to help get the patient back to a normal lifestyle as quickly as possible. In addition, appropriate rehabilitation exercise encourages pet owners to work with their pet daily, improving function and allowing early recognition of a complication, if it arises.

Fracture repair with external coaptation is not optimal because it leads to the degeneration of soft tissue in the affected limb and does not allow access to the site of injury for assessment and rehabilitation modalities. In cases in which external coaptation is the only option for fracture fixation, clients and veterinarians should be aware that degeneration will occur. Limb immobilization leads to loss of articular cartilage strength and density,[34,35] decreased tendon and ligament strength,[34,36] and degenerative joint changes similar to those seen in osteoarthritis. Casting a limb in flexion seems to have fewer deleterious effects on the joints and surroundings structures[34] but means less weight bearing and likely leads to a greater loss of bone density and muscle atrophy.

After the correction of a limb fracture, rehabilitation should initially focus on reducing pain and keeping the patient comfortable and mobile. Initial modalities should include cryotherapy, therapeutic laser, gentle massage, passive range of motion, and gentle weight-bearing exercises. If weight bearing is not attainable in the first several days, pain management should be adjusted to make the patient more comfortable. Cryotherapy can be given immediately after injury or surgery, assuming the patient has and is able to maintain a normal body temperature. Within 24 hours of the injury the affected limb can be taken through gentle passive range of motion, taking great care not to further injure the patient or cause discomfort. Within 12 to 24 hours, the patient should be assisted into a normal standing position to encourage weight bearing, even if it is minimal, on its affected limb. The patient should be encouraged to eat at this time, which helps it to learn that it is able to function on its own.

As the patient progresses through recovery, the prescription for therapeutic exercise can be updated regularly taking care not to push the patient too quickly and always ensuring that those working with the patient understand that if some treatment modality causes significant discomfort it should not be continued. With progress, patients can begin to perform exercises that emphasize active range of motion, in which they are encouraged to flex and extend their joints actively. Examples of exercises that accentuate range of motion are stepping over an obstacle or reaching out for a treat. Focus should also be placed on strengthening of the affected limb and improving proprioception to prevent further injury at this stage of recovery.

Avian patients should be gradually reintroduced to their normal perching habits as a component of their therapeutic exercise. Perches should initially be low and made over a padded landing, such as towels or pillows. Once the bird is able to demonstrate safe mounting and dismounting, an injury becomes less likely.

Patients that have their injured part placed in a cast or immobilized need to participate in controlled activity and therapeutic exercise until they regain normal function and strength. These patients are at a higher risk of injury because of atrophy and contracture,[34] so they are at a much higher risk for reinjury initially.

Neurologic Injuries

In the case of neurologic injuries, there are a variety of presentations stemming from a variety of underlying causes. Spinal trauma, peripheral nerve damage, neuropathic pain related to a prior injury, toxic insult, or infectious diseases can incite neurologic signs in zoologic companion animals. It is important to identify and treat the underlying cause of the disease because managing pain and performing rehabilitation are not as helpful in the face of a progressive disease such as infection, neoplasia, or continued toxin exposure.

Neurologic recovery assisted by rehabilitation can be rewarding but requires patience from the pet owner and veterinarian. Nerve tissue heals slowly, and recovery depends on the cause and severity of the inciting problem. Zoologic companion animals are often affected by trauma, but the basic principles described in this article apply to neurologic deficits resulting from many disease processes. Neurologic injuries can induce neuropathic pain, which can be life threatening and must be dealt with quickly and aggressively to prevent self-trauma[15] and other pain-related maladies.

As with orthopedic injuries, it is essential to ensure that pain is being managed well immediately after the injury with pharmaceutical interventions, acupuncture, and rehabilitation modalities targeted to reduce pain. Such management is the best way to reduce the risk of developing neuropathic pain in later stages of recovery. Rehabilitation modalities used at this stage are similar to those used immediately after an orthopedic injury and include cryotherapy, therapeutic laser, passive range of motion exercise, and gentle massage, if possible. Another essential component of rehabilitation in the early stages of neurologic injury is simulated or assisted weight bearing on the affected limbs. Performing an assisted stand, whether in a bird, small mammal, or reptile, should be done frequently after injury to limit neurogenic muscle loss and retrain the nervous system for standing. The patient must be helped into a normal anatomic standing position, and support should be decreased to make the patient bear as much of its own weight as possible. Eventually the animal weakens and is no longer able to support itself, but the process encourages rebuilding muscle and reestablishing muscle memory. This exercise can seem frustrating in the early stages and it can be tempting to give up, but perseverance often yields good results. As the patient progresses, it can be encouraged to walk with assistance, using manual support or a sling made from a towel or piece of bed linen.

An additional consideration for patients with neurologic injuries is the possibility of self-inflicted trauma because of absent sensation, abnormal sensation, or neuropathic pain. Self-trauma can be problematic in small mammals and birds, so vigilant monitoring is especially important in these species. Pet owners should be instructed to inspect their injured pet daily for scrapes, cuts, or other injuries that may require medical attention. If patients are unable to turn or right themselves, it is important to provide a comfortable supportive bed and turn them regularly to avoid discomfort and pressure sores.

Head Trauma and Head Tilt

Head tilt is a common problem in many species for a variety of reasons. Birds may develop a head tilt secondary to head trauma, whereas it is a common condition in rabbits and chinchillas with otitis media or otitis interna.[37] A head tilt can be uncomfortable and debilitating for patients of all species. Rehabilitating a patient with a head tilt greatly improves the quality of life by improving functionality and reducing discomfort associated with a head tilt.

Patients with a head tilt have severe discomfort in their cervical and cranial thoracic paraspinal muscles as a result of the abnormal head position. These muscle groups should be a major target for therapeutic laser and massage because loosening them and making them more comfortable allows patients to begin changing their head position as they gain the neurologic ability. Gentle cervical passive range of motion and subtle traction is also indicated if cervical trauma and instability have been ruled out. Bringing patients through this gentle range of motion allows cervical vertebrae to articulate normally, preventing muscle contracture and maintaining a normal range of motion while the patient is recovering. Traction provides axial elongation of the spine, which further supports a normal range of motion, but can cause spinal cord or vascular damage if excessive force is applied.[38] For the patient with a chronic head tilt, application of an appropriately heated warm pack can aid in range of motion activities and make massage more comfortable.

Assisted standing progressing to assisted walking is important for these patients because their head tilt may be so severe that they cannot stand or perch normally, which may alter their ability to eat, drink, and sleep, so it is important to take these factors into consideration. As with other neurologic injuries, patients should be assisted into a normal anatomic stance and supported only as much as they require. These patients often need abundant support initially, but as they improve they are able to do more and more on their own.

SUMMARY

It is vital to assess the underlying cause for injury or illness in zoologic companion animals, just as it is in other species. Once the underlying condition has been identified and appropriate treatment is instituted, the recovery process begins. Pain management is an essential component of physical rehabilitation because it leads to better patient compliance, more rapid recovery, and more ethical veterinary practice. Rehabilitation techniques are designed for improving recovery from injury or trauma and can also be used to improve quality of life in patients with ongoing or progressive medical conditions. Rehabilitation provides patients, pet owners, and veterinarians a gentle positive experience that leaves the patient less painful and more functional.

REFERENCES

1. Gaynor JS, Muir WW. Handbook of veterinary pain management. 2nd edition. St Louis (MO): Elsevier; 2009. p. 467–506.
2. Heinrichs K. Superficial thermal modalities. In: Millis DL, Levine D, Taylor RA, editors. Canine rehabilitation and physical therapy. St Louis (MO): Saunders; 2004. p. 277–88.
3. Scapigliati G, Buonocore F, Maini M. Biological activity of cytokines: an evolutionary perspective. Curr Pharm Des 2006;12(24):3071–81.

4. Pare JA, Sigler L, Rosenthal KL, et al. Microbiology: fungal and bacterial diseases of reptiles. In: Mader DR, editor. Reptile medicine and surgery. 2nd edition. St Louis (MO): Saunders; 2006. p. 217–38.
5. Wright KM. Overview of amphibian medicine. In: Mader DR, editor. Reptile medicine and surgery. 2nd edition. St Louis (MO): Saunders; 2006. p. 941–71.
6. Pereira MCMC, de Pinho CB, Medrado ARP, et al. Influence of 670 nm low-level laser therapy on mast cells and vascular response of cutaneous injuries. J Photochem Photobiol B 2010;98(3):188–92.
7. Zhang LX, Tong XJ, Yuan XH, et al. Effects of 660 nm gallium-aluminum-arsenide low-energy laser on nerve regeneration after acellular nerve allograft in rats. Synapse 2010;64:152–60.
8. Barbosa RI, Marcolino AM, de Jesus Guirro RR, et al. Comparative effects of wavelengths of low-power laser in regeneration of sciatic nerve in rats following crushing lesion. Lasers Med Sci 2010;25:423–30.
9. Pejcic A, Kojovic D, Kesic L, et al. The effects of low level laser irradiation on gingival inflammation. Photomed Laser Surg 2010;28(1):69–74.
10. Liu XG, Zhou YJ, Liu TC, et al. Effects of low-level laser irradiation on rat skeletal muscle injury after eccentric exercise. Photomed Laser Surg 2009;27(6):863–9.
11. Venezian GC, da Silva MA, Maetto RG, et al. Low level laser effects on pain to palpation and electromyographic activity in TMD patients: a double-blind, randomized, placebo-controlled study. Cranio 2010;28(2):84–91.
12. Dirican A, Andacogluc O, Johnson R, et al. The short-term effects of low-level laser therapy in the management of breast-cancer-related lymphedema. Support Care Cancer 2010 May 6. [Epub ahead of print].
13. Busnardo VL, Biondo-Simoes ML. [Effects of low-level helium-neon laser on induced wound healing in rats]. Rev Bras Fisioter 2010;14(1):45–51 [in Portuguese].
14. Maluf AP, Maluf RP, Brito Cda R, et al. Mechanical evaluation of the influence of low-level laser therapy in secondary stability of implants in mice shinbones. Lasers Med Sci 2010;25(5):693–8.
15. Pires-Oliveira DAA, Oliveira RF, Amadei SU, et al. Laser 904 nm action on bone repair in rats with osteoporosis. Osteoporos Int 2010 Mar 4. [Epub ahead of print].
16. Shaver SL, Robinson NG, Wright BD, et al. A multimodal approach to pain management of suspected neuropathic pain in a prairie falcon (*Falco mexicanus*). J Avian Med Surg 2009;23(3):209–13.
17. Hamilton S, Millis DL, Taylor RA, et al. Therapeutic exercises. In: Millis DL, Levine D, Taylor RA, editors. Canine rehabilitation and physical therapy. St Louis (MO): Saunders; 2004. p. 244–63.
18. McMillan MW, Whitaker KE, Hughes D, et al. Effect of body position on the arterial partial pressures of oxygen and carbon dioxide in spontaneously breathing, conscious dogs in an intensive care unit. J Vet Emerg Crit Care(San Antonio) 2009;19(6):564–70.
19. Hoste EAJ, Roosens CDVK, Bracke S, et al. Acute effects of upright position on gas exchange in patients with acute respiratory distress syndrome. J Intensive Care Med 2005;20(1):43–9.
20. Roanski EA, Bedenice D, Lofgren J, et al. The effect of body position, sedation and thoracic bandaging on functional residual capacity in healthy deep-chested dogs. Can J Vet Res 2010;74:34–9.
21. Martin HD, Ritchie BW. Orthopedic surgical techniques. In: Ritchie BW, Harrison GJ, Harrison LW, editors. Avian medicine: principles and applications. Lake Worth (FL): Wingers Publishing; 1994. p. 1137–69.

22. Degernes LA, Lind PJ, Olson DE, et al. Evaluating avian fractures for use of methylmethacrylate orthopedic technique. J Assoc Avian Vet 1989;3(2):64–7.
23. Cooney J, Mueller L. Postoperative management of the avian orthopedic patient. Semin Avian Exotic Pet Med 1994;3(2):100–7.
24. Lane E, Latham T. Managing pain using heat and cold therapy. Paediatr Nurs 2009;21(6):14–8.
25. Steiss JE, McCauley L. Therapeutic ultrasound. In: Millis DL, Levine D, Taylor RA, editors. Canine rehabilitation and physical therapy. St Louis (MO): Saunders; 2004. p. 324–36.
26. Wimsatt J, Dressen P, Dennison C, et al. Ultrasound therapy for the prevention and correction of contractures and bone mineral loss associated with wing bandaging in the domestic pigeon (Columba livia). J Zoo Wildl Med 2000; 31(2):190–5.
27. Le Blanc-Louvry I, Costaglioli B, Boulon C, et al. Does mechanical massage of the abdominal wall after colectomy reduce postoperative pain and shorten the duration of ileus? Results of a randomized study. J Gastrointest Surg 2002; 6(1):43–9.
28. Field T, Diego M, Hernandez-Reif M. Moderate pressure is essential for massage therapy effects. Int J Neurosci 2010;120:381–5.
29. Diego MA, Field T, Hernandez-Reif M, et al. Preterm infant massage elicits consistent increases in vagal activity and gastric motility that are associated with greater weight gain. Acta Paediatr 2007;96(11):1588–91.
30. Diego MA, Field T, Hernandez-Reif M. Vagal activity, gastric motility, and weight gain in massaged preterm neonates. J Pediatr 2005;147(1):50–5.
31. Huang SY, Santo MD, Wadden KP, et al. Short-duration massage at the hamstrings musculotendinous junction induces greater range of motion. J Strength Cond Res 2010;24(7):1917–24.
32. Donoyama N, Shibasaki M. Differences in practitioners' proficiency affect the effectiveness of massage therapy on physical and psychological states. J Bodyw Mov Ther 2010;14(3):239–44.
33. Albertin A, Kerppers II, Amorim CF, et al. The effect of manual therapy on masseter muscle pain and spasm. Electromyogr Clin Neurophysiol 2010; 50(2):107–12.
34. Millis DL. Responses of musculoskeletal tissues to disuse and remobilization. In: Millis DL, Levine D, Taylor RA, editors. Canine rehabilitation and physical therapy. St Louis (MO): Saunders; 2004. p. 113–53.
35. Jortikka MO, Inkinen RI, Tammi MI, et al. Immobilisation causes longlasting matrix changes both in immobilised and contralateral joint cartilage. Ann Rheum Dis 1997;56:225–61.
36. Yasuda K, Hayashi K. Changes in biomechanical properties of tendons and ligaments from joint disuse. Osteoarthr Cartil 1999;7:122–9.
37. Deeb BJ, Carpenter JW. Neurologic and musculoskeletal diseases. In: Quesenberry KE, Carpenter JW, editors. Ferrets, rabbits, and rodents clinical medicine and surgery. 2nd edition. St Louis (MO): Saunders; 2004. p. 203–10.
38. Martinez-Lage JF, Almagro MJ, Izura V, et al. Cervical spinal cord infarction after posterior fossa surgery: a case-based update. Childs Nerv Syst 2009;25(12): 1541–6.

Acupuncture for Zoological Companion Animals

Marilyn A. Koski, DVM[a,b],*

KEYWORDS

- Zoological companion animal • Acupuncture
- Traditional Chinese veterinary medicine • Analgesia

Veterinarians increasingly are asked by clients to advise them on the efficacy of complementary and alternative veterinary medical therapies for the treatment of their pets. Research in the human and veterinary medical fields of complementary and alternative medicine (CAM) has increased dramatically in recent years, and as a result clients are more aware of these treatment modalities either as the result of direct experience or via exposure to the literature and media. A 1993 article in the *New England Journal of Medicine* estimates that 1 in 3 adults uses some form of unconventional medicine and 70% of those patients do so without the advice or knowledge of their primary care practitioners.[1,2] The investigators suggest that the lack of communication between practitioner and patient exists because most physicians have little understanding of alternative therapies. Veterinarians are facing a similar situation, and we would be wise to learn from our physician colleagues and strive toward better client communication by gaining a general understanding of the basic principles of common complementary and alternative veterinary medical therapies.

Critics of CAM and complementary and alternative veterinary medicine (CAVM) often cite desperation, lack of knowledge, or misguided goals as the reasons veterinary clients and human patients pursue alternative therapies.[3] The fear of the outcome of serious diseases, feelings of helplessness, and the hope for cure or relief of pain are reasons that veterinary clients and human patients seek both conventional and alternative medical therapies.[3] Not all conventional therapies are supported by in-depth studies, and many times outcomes of accepted conventional treatments do not yield

The author has nothing to disclose.
[a] Companion Avian and Exotic Pet Medicine Wellness Service, University of California, Veterinary Medical Teaching Hospital, One Shields Avenue, Davis, CA 95616-8747, USA
[b] Small and Exotic Animal Acupuncture Service, University of California, Veterinary Medical Teaching Hospital, One Shields Avenue, Davis, CA 95616-8747, USA
* Companion Avian and Exotic Pet Medicine Wellness Service, University of California, Veterinary Medical Teaching Hospital, One Shields Avenue, Davis, CA 95616-8747.
E-mail address: makoski@vmth.ucdavis.edu

the results physicians and veterinarians hope for, yet these are offered as treatment options. Experimental surgeries and therapies are often recommended based on limited experience in situations where scientific evidence is not available, yet many medical professionals will omit alternative therapies for reasons of limited scientific evidence. Medical professionals may evaluate the efficacy of a therapy based on experience, but a causal relationship should not be established by clinical experience alone.

CAVM includes a wide range of therapies including acupuncture, herbal medicine, chiropractic, tui na (pronounced twee-na), massage, food therapy (nutrition), and homeopathy. A veterinarian cannot be expected to be well versed on all CAVM modalities, but a basic knowledge of the most available and most scientifically researched therapies is helpful, in addition to establishing professional relationships with local veterinary practitioners trained in CAVM modalities to facilitate referrals.

Wynn and Wolpe[3] present a workable model of ethical considerations when considering alternative therapies for a veterinary patient, adapted from a human model presented by Adams and colleagues.[4] Wynn and Wolpe recommend first assessing the severity and acuteness of the illness, and then evaluating the potential for cure using evidence-based treatment. Next, the conventional treatment should be compared with the alternative treatment with regard to invasiveness and toxicity. Third, the quality and legitimacy of the evidence for efficacy and safety of the alternative therapy is evaluated. Lastly, ethical use of CAVM depends on the client's level of comprehension of all aspects of the alternative therapy, including risks and cost.

The report of CAM therapies generated by the Institute of Medicine (IOM) at the National Academy of Sciences in 2005 presented a virtually identical format for human patient assessment when considering alternative treatment. The report noted that the goal should be the provision of comprehensive medical care that is based on the best scientific evidence available regarding benefits and harm, which encourages patients to share in decision making about therapeutic options, and that promotes choices in care that can include CAM therapies when appropriate.[5,6] The report stated that appropriate, comprehensive medical care included "suspending any categorical disbelief in CAM therapies".[6]

Acupuncture represents the most commonly practiced and extensively researched of all the CAM and CAVM modalities. It is considered a valid therapeutic mode of treatment that can be integrated into Western veterinary medicine for the treatment of large, small and zoological companion animal patients.[1,2,7-9]

LEGALITY AND TRAINING (IN THE UNITED STATES)

In 2007, the American Veterinary Medical Association (AVMA) presented guidelines on CAVM in its AVMA directory and resource manual.[10] These guidelines stated that the use of CAVM was in accordance with the practice of veterinary medicine, and that veterinarians who choose to use CAVM techniques should acquire the requisite skills and education to perform these treatment modalities. The guidelines also stated that all veterinary medicine, including CAVM, should be held to the same standards, and that claims of safety and efficacy should be proven by the scientific method.

In most states in the United States veterinary acupuncture must be performed by a licensed veterinarian, but there are presently no regulations ensuring the competence of a veterinary acupuncturist. Specialized courses and certification training in veterinary acupuncture are offered at several institutions in the United States:

- Chi Institute, Gainesville, Florida (www.tcvm.com)
- International Veterinary Acupuncture Society (IVAS), Fort Collins, Colorado (Ivasoffice@aol.com)

- Medical Acupuncture for Veterinarians at Colorado State University, Fort Collins, Colorado, contact Colorado Veterinary Medical Association (CVMA) at 303 318 0447 or email info@colovma.org.

Programs at these institutions offer veterinarians intensive training in the theory and technique of small and large animal acupuncture. Zoological companion animal veterinarians who consider referring patients to a veterinary acupuncturist are advised to inquire as to the individual's training and experience. This article will hopefully serve as a guide for the zoological companion animal practitioner who is considering either incorporating complementary medicine into his or her practice, or referring patients to an acupuncturist.

DEFINITION OF ACUPUNCTURE

The word acupuncture is derived from the 2 Latin words *acus*, needle and *pungere*, to pierce or prick. Acupuncture involves the use of solid, extremely fine, needles to diagnose, treat, and prevent disease by stimulating the body's own ability to heal. Hypodermic needles can create some of the same effects of acupuncture therapy, but because of the relatively large diameter, their use can cause more local tissue damage. The goal of acupuncture is to create the least amount of trauma to the body while eliciting the greatest beneficial effect.[11] The use of fine, solid needles is referred to as dry needle acupuncture (**Fig. 1**), while other related techniques may involve injection of small amounts of fluid, aquapuncture, and the use of electrical stimulation on acupuncture needles called electroacupuncture, to name a few. The aquapuncture technique uses a fluid (eg, vitamin B12 or saline) to create prolonged stimulation at an acupuncture site, or in situations where the patient will not tolerate retention of a dry needle for any period of time. Electroacupuncture is used to enhance neuromodulation and stimulate the release of different neurochemicals through variation of electrical frequency and duration of treatment.

There are more than 80 different acupuncture techniques in China alone, with additional methods practiced in Korea, Japan, Europe, Vietnam, and the Americas. The various techniques share a similar diagnostic and therapeutic approach, but there is no universal "traditional Chinese acupuncture," just as Western medicine is interpreted and practiced differently throughout the world despite its shared principles and theories.[12]

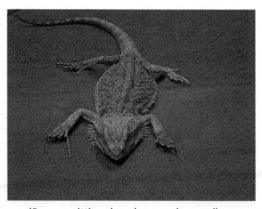

Fig. 1. Bearded dragon (*Pogona vitticeps*) undergoes dry needle acupuncture therapy.

HISTORY OF ACUPUNCTURE

The precise origin of acupuncture is still debated, but evidence exists that acupuncture was practiced as long as 5000 years ago, and not solely in China.[11] The Egyptian medical treatises of 1550 BC made reference to acupuncture-like treatments, and there is a Hindu reference to acupuncture in the Aveda scriptures dated 1300 BC. South African Bantu tribesmen and North American Eskimos used sharp bones and stones to scratch parts of their bodies to treat disease. Evidence suggests that acupuncture developed throughout the world both by demonstration and description among individuals, and also spontaneously among people who did not experience cultural cross-over. The well-preserved remains of a man in the Tyrolean Alps, dated more than 5000 years old, revealed evidence of a skin-piercing technique resembling a form of acupuncture, suggesting the use of acupuncture in Central Europe around 3200 BC.[13,14]

Chinese acupuncture dates back more than 2500 years, with the first veterinary acupuncture text, Bai-Li's Canon of Veterinary Medicine, written in 620 BC.[15] The Chinese developed acupuncture techniques as one part of a much larger and multifaceted system of medicine referred to as Traditional Chinese Medicine (TCM) for humans and Traditional Chinese Veterinary Medicine (TCVM) for animals. For the sake of simplicity, contemporary acupuncture can be described as either traditional Chinese medical acupuncture or Western medical acupuncture (also referred to as transpositional acupuncture in veterinary medicine).[16,17]

Traditional Chinese acupuncture originated from agrarian and environmental roots, where health is determined by metaphysical concepts of energy flow within the body and the effects of the surrounding environment. The traditional Chinese acupuncture system describes good health on the basis of a balance between opposite forces (Yin and Yang) and the flow of energy, "life force" or *qi* (also spelled *chi*, both pronounced "chee").[16]

It is thought that *qi* flows along definite paths or "meridians" in the body, and disease conditions represent a blockage or disruption of flow of this energy. Disease assessment is based on detailed observational clues including tongue appearance, mental attitude, the appearance and odor of feces and urine, palpation of painful areas or trigger points on the body, and overall body condition (eg, integument, nails, posture, and muscle tone). The ancient Chinese also described in great detail the different pulse qualities they felt at arterial loci, and they believed that these variations in pulsation points were caused by alterations in *qi*. The most commonly presented theory of TCM/TCVM is based on energetic, not anatomic, concepts.[2]

It is extremely challenging for most present-day health care providers to embrace the traditional Chinese theory and its complex, though elegant, metaphysical concepts, as they clash so strongly with mainstream Western medicine and its contemporary scientific disciplines such as anatomy, biochemistry, physiology, and pharmacology.[7]

It is important that some scholars believe that the interpretation of TCM/TCVM as being a metaphysical- and energetic-based medicine is incorrect, and that this conceptual error is due, in part, to poor translation of the early Chinese texts. These scholars believe that ancient Chinese acupuncturists, lacking the diagnostic and anatomic insight and technologies we have today, described the vascular and peripheral neurologic system using the best descriptive vernacular available to them within the context of their daily lives. Some argue that if ancient Chinese acupuncturists were afforded the same technology and understanding of anatomy and physiology that we have today, they would have described acupuncture theory and practice using the same terminology and perspective we ascribe to contemporary Western acupuncture.[18,19] The ancient Chinese body maps depicting acupuncture points and *qi* meridians closely follow arterial and neurologic pathways. Some medical professionals believe that it is only logical to view acupuncture from a purely neurophysiologic basis and to discard all traditional Chinese theories of acupuncture. To discard more than 3000 years of empirical evidence seems equally illogical, when these extensive empirical observations may provide a useful guide to future research and understanding of acupuncture mechanisms.

Western acupuncture medicine has its basis in anatomy and physiology, with emphasis on the concept of trigger points, and neuroanatomy. The Western medical approach to acupuncture can provide an intelligible bridge for Western-trained medical professionals to allow the integration of acupuncture into their treatment regimes.

During the 1960s interest in acupuncture medicine increased in the West, with a dramatic upswing after Nixon's visit to China in the 1971. Americans were exposed to acupuncture via news reports and film. This new interest in TCM/TCVM allowed freer exchange of ideas, and veterinary professionals sought ways to incorporate the use of acupuncture into their practices. The Western veterinary approach to acupuncture, also referred to as "transpositional" acupuncture, developed at this time.[17] Ancient Chinese veterinary acupuncture point body maps existed only for cows, pigs, horses, and poultry, but these illustrated few acupuncture points with imprecise locations. In the 1970s in North America, veterinarians invited human acupuncturists from various parts of the world to assist them in devising point maps for dogs and cats using human point system maps as a template. Due to postural differences and variations in anatomy among animal species, placement of points did not correlate easily with human anatomy and point maps. The tail, for example, when it exists, represents an additional area for acupuncture stimulation that has no analogous site on the human body.

One method being used presently to resolve the problem of accurate point transposition from humans to animals involves identifying the neurovascular structures, peripheral nerve locations, and central nervous system associations to acupuncture points in humans. As neuroanatomical research of acupuncture points progresses and more of these correlations are made, veterinary acupuncturists will be able to identify the same anatomic structures on animals and thus be able to identify the location of the analogous human point.

Even more valuable to the advancement of veterinary acupuncture is the neuroanatomical research of acupuncture points being conducted directly on animal species. Ongoing research at the Colorado State University of Veterinary Medicine and the University of Veterinary Medicine in Florida is directed toward the creation of accurate transposition point location maps for the dog, cat, and horse.[20–22] To date, no comprehensive neuroanatomically accurate acupuncture point atlases exist for nonhuman species.[20,23]

MECHANISM OF ACTION

Although traditional Chinese and Western veterinary medical acupuncture theories differ, successful treatment is based on the same requirement: selection of effective acupuncture points or acupoints.[12] In traditional Chinese veterinary medical acupuncture, an acupoint is referred to as *Shu Xue* (pronounced shoo-shway, where *Shu* means transporting, distributing, communicating, and *Xue* means depression, hole, outlet). The acupoint is considered a hole in the skin that communicates with internal organs via a channel or meridian.[15] There are 361 classic acupoints associated with meridians, and more than 2000 extrameridian acupoints recognized in the ancient Chinese literature. Contemporary research has shown that 309 of these acupoints are located on or near nerves, and 286 acupoints are surrounded by small nerve bundles in close proximity to major blood vessels.[12,24]

The physiologic effects of acupuncture are the result of neuromodulation occurring from direct nerve stimulation.[23] The needling of tissue at an acupuncture point causes activation of the peripheral nervous system, which results in responses from the peripheral, autonomic and central nervous system.[11,12,25] Acupuncture causes neurohumoral and neuroendocrine changes that alter pain transmission and aid the body's intrinsic pain control mechanisms.[25]

The tingling, achy, or numb feeling noted by human patients receiving acupuncture is referred to as de qi (pronounced duh-chee or de-chee), and it is considered crucial by many to yield the best therapeutic effect. The variation in de qi sensation is thought to be the result of stimulation of the different types of afferent nerve fibers (II, III, or unmyelinated IV).[12,26,27]

Of the myriad effects acupuncture has on the body, analgesia has been the most scrutinized and is most represented in the literature. The precise mechanisms to describe acupuncture's effects are still under debate, but a growing body of evidence demonstrates that acupuncture analgesia has physiologic, anatomic, and neurochemical bases.[26] The dominant theory states that acupuncture (especially electroacupuncture) promotes analgesia via stimulation of certain receptor sites in the dorsal horn of the spinal cord, resulting in the release of neurochemicals such as β-endorphins, enkephalins, and serotonin.[28–32] Numerous studies involving humans and animals have demonstrated that electroacupuncture at various intensities is capable of producing analgesia owing to the release of different brain neuropeptides.[28,29,33] Peripheral stimulation of large sensory afferent nerves using electroacupuncture modulates nociceptive input into the spinal cord, producing analgesia following the "Gate Control Theory".[12]

Additional animal research revealed that acupuncture changes opioidergic and monoaminergic neurotransmission activity in the brainstem, thalamus, hypothalamus, and/or pituitary.[34,35] Clinical research also supports that acupuncture's effects are mediated through regulation of the autonomic nervous system. A study of irritable bladder symptoms in humans revealed improvement in detrusor (urinary bladder) muscle function equal in effect to standard drug therapy with oxybutynin.[36]

In 1997, Pomeranz[30] presented 17 lines of experimental evidence to support the neurophysiologic mechanism of acupuncture analgesia. A few key points from the extensive evidence he presented include: successful acupuncture requires an intact and functioning nervous system; the effects of acupuncture can be blocked by many opiate antagonists and by antibodies to endorphins (suggesting that acupuncture works partially via the release of endogenous endorphins); and individuals who share cerebrospinal fluid or blood via cross-circulation conditions show changes when only one of the individuals is needled.

Acupuncture has also been shown to inhibit inflammation, in part by activation of the hypothalamic-pituitary-adrenal axis, to increase circulation to muscle tissue and enhance nitric oxide generation, and to improve wound healing.[37,38] Acupuncture has been shown, in numerous species, to affect gastric and colonic motility and have antiemetic activity in humans associated with postoperative and postchemotherapy nausea/vomiting.[39–41]

The most promising research investigating acupuncture's mechanism of action involves the use of contemporary neuroimaging techniques such as functional magnetic resonance imaging, positron emission tomography, electroencephalography, and magnetoencephalography. These imaging modalities provide a safe method for monitoring brain activity while trying to map the neural correlates of acupuncture.[35,42,43]

The use of certain drugs (eg, opioids, glucocorticoids, benzodiazepines) has been shown to potentially enhance or interfere with the effects of acupuncture.[44–47] If acupuncture is to be integrated into a patient's treatment plan that includes the use of these medications, the acupuncturist and zoological companion animal practitioner should discuss where adjustments should be made to maximize the potential for combined therapies.

Safety

Acupuncture, if administered by a trained and experienced acupuncturist, does not pose a significant risk to the patient. In human acupuncture medicine serious complications have been described, but their occurrence is exceedingly rare.[48,49] The National Institutes of Health Consensus Statement states "one of the advantages of acupuncture is that the incidence of adverse effects is substantially lower than many of the drugs or other accepted procedures for the same conditions."[50] Prospective studies examining the incidence of adverse effects of acupuncture in humans have been conducted covering a variety of countries in a range of clinical conditions. A review of these studies revealed the rate of serious adverse effects to be 3 per million treatments, which is much less than many conventional medical treatments.[51]

Acupuncture should be used with caution in patients who are pregnant, have severe blood coagulopathies, are severely debilitated, or who are extremely febrile, while the use of electroacupuncture is contraindicated in all these patients. Electroacupuncture should also be avoided in patients with seizure disorders, severe local skin infections, and local malignancies.[25] Acupuncture needles should never be placed directly in neoplastic or infected tissue, or directly in open wounds.

An important consideration for the zoological companion animal practitioner who contemplates referring a patient for acupuncture is the acupuncturist's experience with zoological companion animals. If the acupuncturist is not familiar with the species to be referred, it may be possible for the acupuncturist to come to the practice of the zoological companion animal practitioner and provide the acupuncture service. This type of joint appointment can enhance the rapport between the zoological companion animal practitioner and the acupuncturist, as they both gain a better understanding of each other's specialty As this working relationship evolves and potential applications for acupuncture are realized, a more integrated approach to zoological animal veterinary care can result. Clients are often very appreciative of this cooperative approach because it emphasizes their veterinarian's devotion to their pet, a willingness to provide services beyond the scope of the clinic, and an open-minded attitude to patient care.

Pain in Zoological Companion Animals

Although an understanding of acupuncture's analgesic mechanism of action has advanced in recent years, most of the information is based on research using mice, rats, rabbits, nonhuman primates, dogs, and humans. Although similarities in neuroanatomy and physiology among animal species allow some extrapolation of information, many of our zoological companion animal species are unique, and comparisons cannot easily be made.

A further complication to species comparison exists in the area of pain recognition. The lack of a gold standard for pain assessment seriously hampers our ability to evaluate pain in zoological companion animal patients, and consequently to accurately judge the responses to analgesic acupuncture techniques. In 2002, an international, multidisciplinary workshop composed of 29 experts in animal and human pain was held to discuss the comparative aspects of pain research and treatment. One of the results of this meeting was the creation of a consensus statement identifying the need for a cross-species approach to the study of animal pain.[52] This consensus statement represents a call to action, intended to motivate human and veterinary medical professionals to communicate and collaborate in a cross-disciplinary manner in order to advance the study of pain in animals and humans.

Unique Aspects of Zoological Companion Animal Acupuncture

Behavioral aspects

The use of acupuncture in our zoological companion animal species presents unique challenges when compared with its use in domestic large and small mammals, but its potential for benefit is significant. Many of our zoological companion animal patients are inherently fractious and infrequently handled; as a result, they are less amenable to calming through tactile or vocal assurance than our domestic dogs and cats. In addition, many of our zoological companion animal patients are prey species who are wary of unfamiliar sensations and environmental situations. It is very important to assess the potential stress applied by any technique and consider whether the potential benefits outweigh the risks. In the hands of a competent acupuncturist who is familiar with the behavior and temperament of zoological companion animal species, acupuncture treatments can be tailored to the needs of the individual.

The excitable and highly energetic personality of most birds may impose the need for more physical restraint and greater practitioner patience to ensure the safe and effective administration of acupuncture. Psittacine birds may tolerate restraint for dry needle therapy if the owner is present to soothe and stroke the patient. Another approach that is effective with birds is to dim the lights until they are almost completely off, place the needles quickly, and have the bird remain within audible range of the owner's voice. Raptorial species that are accustomed to jesses and hoods will often readily accept dry needle acupuncture without restraint.

Small mammal patients such as rabbits, chinchillas, and guinea pigs are often very amenable to acupuncture therapy when provided a quiet and secure environment for treatment (**Fig. 2**). These patients tolerate dry needle treatments best when the needles are placed quickly and then the patient is released from restraint. The author prefers to allow rabbit patients to ambulate freely on a clinic floor, with access to food and interaction with companions, all the while with needles in place. Similarly, chelonian patients can sometimes be placed on platforms that prevent their limbs to contact the ground, and dry needles can be safely placed while they "ambulate" in midair (**Fig. 3**). Ferrets, rats, and mice can be more challenging patients, due to their energetic personalities and their inherent agility. Special attention needs to be paid to the ferret acupuncture patient because of its predisposition to investigation with its mouth and potential risk of foreign body (needle) ingestion.

Aquapuncture (the injection of minute amounts of sterile saline, injectable B vitamins, and so forth) can be used initially in specific calming acupoints to promote relaxation before the placement of the remaining needles. For highly stressed or hyperactive patients, the technique of aquapuncture may be used for the entire treatment, to deliver stimulation to the various acupoints quickly and to allow the fluid to provide the prolonged nerve activation usually created by longer duration of dry needle placement. The author has used the aquapuncture technique in many highly active ferrets, with good results.

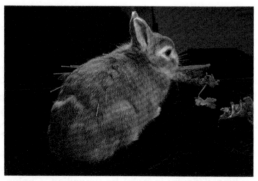

Fig. 2. Dry needle acupuncture treatment on a dwarf rabbit. (*Courtesy of* Don Preisler, UC Davis School of Veterinary Medicine, Davis, CA.)

A common benefit of acupuncture noted among humans and nonhuman patients alike is the sedating and almost tranquilizing effect acupuncture can promote. Many veterinary patients may appear nervous or reluctant during their initial acupuncture session, but they gradually relax and often fall asleep as the session progresses. It is thought that the release of mood-altering neurotransmitters produced by the needle

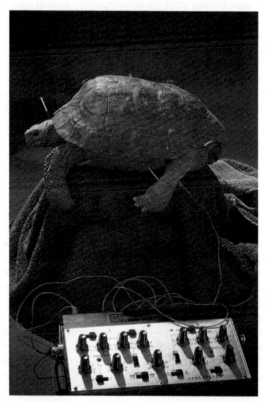

Fig. 3. Desert tortoise (*Gopherus agassizzii*), on suspended platform, undergoes both dry needle and electroacupuncture therapy. (*Courtesy of* Don Preisler, UC Davis School of Veterinary Medicine, Davis, CA.)

stimulation may be the cause of this response. This effect creates a rewarding scenario for the patient, client, and veterinarian, when treatments are a positive and relaxed experience.

Anatomic aspects

As previously stated, there are no comprehensive, neuroanatomically accurate acupuncture point maps for nonhuman species; some limited point guides have been presented. Drs Schoen, Partington, and Ferguson have described limited acupuncture point guides for avian species based on empirical point transposition and interpretation from ancient Chinese poultry acupoint charts.[15,53,54]

One of the most stunning obstacles we confront when using acupuncture in zoological companion species relates to the extreme anatomic diversity among the species and the resulting difficulty in point transposition. Chelonians, for example, with their carapace and plastron, limit the use of acupuncture sites to the limbs, head, and tail. Snakes present the opposite dilemma, with easy access to vertebral associated points and no options for extremity acupuncture points. In some species of reptiles, boney cutaneous plates and excessively thick skin create considerable barriers to acupuncture needle insertion. Avian species also present anatomic challenges to acupuncture treatment. Fusion of the boney skeleton along portions of the limbs (eg, tibiotarsus) and vertebrae (synsacrum and notarium) create problems of point transposition.

Due to the small size of many zoological companion animal species, acupoints are correspondingly small and located in close proximity to one another. Discerning individual points can be unrealistic, and some points may have to be avoided. In addition, the small size of some patients and the delicacy of their skin can pose significant risk of tendon or ligament damage or excessive blood loss when using dry needle or aquapuncture techniques. These tiny patients are best treated with dry needles that are not left in place; instead, a needle is placed in each acupoint and gently manipulated for 10 to 15 seconds, then removed, and a new needle is used to repeat the process in the next acupoint.[15]

Patient Selection for Acupuncture

The author recommends that acupuncture be considered early in the development of a patient's treatment plan and not be relegated to the "last resort" category of treatment options. This perspective is shared by practitioners of both evidence-based veterinary acupuncture and traditional Chinese veterinary medical acupuncturists. The TCVM practitioner views all signs of illness as an imbalance of energy and the longer the imbalance occurs untreated, the more the body progresses toward serious and potentially irreparable dysfunction.[30] From the perspective of the evidence-based acupuncturist, the use of acupuncture as a rescue therapy for terminal patients, such as those in organ failure, exhibiting severe nervous system dysfunction, or in end-stage neoplastic disease, is not appropriate. Acupuncture in these advanced cases may provide analgesia, relaxation, or appetite stimulation, but not cure. Successful acupuncture therapy requires the patient to have an intact functioning nervous system and usually involves multiple treatments.[30] As previously discussed, the use of certain drugs (eg, opioids) must also be considered when incorporating acupuncture into the treatment regimen, as they may interfere with acupuncture's efficacy.[47]

The most common uses for acupuncture in veterinary medicine are in the areas of pain management, geriatric medicine, and sports medicine.[18,55] Some conditions that may be helped by acupuncture include: cervical, thoracolumbar, and lumbosacral hyperpathia; orofacial pain; degenerative joint disease; intervertebral disc pain; perioperative

Table 1 Zoological companion animal conditions commonly considered for acupuncture therapy	
Condition	Example
Musculoskeletal diseases/disorders	Degenerative joint disease (DJD) and osteoarthritis (eg, lumbar vertebral spondylosis in geriatric lagomorphs and osteoarthritis and DJD in guinea pigs secondary to chronic scurvy)
Hind limb paresis	Chelonians, lizards, and avian species: secondary to prolonged gravid status or trauma or disuse
Gastrointestinal disorders	Diarrhea and emesis in ferrets, ileus in lagomorphs, guinea pigs, chinchillas, chelonians, and lizards
Urinary incontinence not caused by bacterial infection or cystic calculi	Geriatric lagomorphs and rodents
Chronic cutaneous conditions	Slow-healing wounds and pruritus in all species, avian feather picking

and postoperative pain; vestibular disease; degenerative myelopathy; chronic visceral hyperalgesia; anorexia; tendon/ligament injuries; chemotherapy-associated emesis; gastrointestinal motility disorders (colic, ileus); asthma; sinusitis; and generalized weakness.[18,25,36,40,56–64]

The clinical research literature devoted to the use of acupuncture in zoological companion animal species is heavily skewed toward rats, mice, rabbits, and (to some degree) ferrets, due to the use of these species in human comparative and veterinary medical research. The specific application of acupuncture to the individual avian, reptile, lagomorph, and rodent patient is represented primarily by anecdotal information and isolated case reports in the literature.[65–68]

The selection of appropriate zoological companion animal patients for acupuncture depends on several criteria, with the most important including the potential stress of the treatment on the patient, the experience of the acupuncturist with the specific species, the nature of the disease to be treated, the client's compliance to an acupuncture treatment schedule, and the feasibility of the treatment goals. Patients being considered for acupuncture should receive individualized treatment plans devised by the zoological companion animal practitioner and the acupuncturist. **Table 1** is a list of conditions common to zoological companion animals, representing a few examples of common conditions that may be identified by owners and veterinarians, and amenable to acupuncture therapy. Acupuncturists do not direct the use of acupuncture to specific conditions but instead treat the whole animal; however, **Table 1** offers the clinician a guide for potential referral to an acupuncturist.

SUMMARY

Human medical and veterinary interest in acupuncture has grown dramatically in recent years, especially in the area of analgesia. The limited evidence-based literature specific to zoological companion animal acupuncture and analgesia emphasizes the need for further research to expand the knowledge and understanding of these unique patients. This article is intended to provide a guide for the zoological companion animal practitioner to gain a basic understanding of acupuncture and its potential for use in the zoological companion animal patient.

REFERENCES

1. Eisenberg DM. Unconventional medicine in the United States: prevalence, costs, and patterns of use. N Engl J Med 1993;328:246–52.
2. Peterson JR. Acupuncture in the 1990s. A review for the primary care physician. Arch Fam Med 1996;5(4):237–40 [discussion: 241].
3. Wynn SG, Wolpe PR. The majority view of ethics and professionalism in alternative medicine. J Am Vet Med Assoc 2005;226(4):516–20.
4. Adams KE, Cohen MH, Eisenberg DM. Ethical considerations of complementary and alternative medical therapies in conventional medical settings. Ann Intern Med 2002;137:660–4.
5. Cohen MH. Legal and ethical issues relating to use of complementary therapies in pediatric hematology/oncology. J Pediatr Hematol Oncol 2006;28(3):190–3.
6. Committee on the use of complementary and alternative medicine by the American Public. Report on use of complementary and alternative medical therapies. Washington DC: Institute of Medicine at the National Academy of Science; 2005.
7. Cheng KJ. Neuroanatomical basis of acupuncture treatment for some common illnesses. Acupunct Med 2009;27(2):61–4.
8. McFarland B, Bigelow D, Zani B, et al. Complementary and alternative medicine use in Canada and the United States. Am J Public Health 2002;92(10):1616–8.
9. Pascoe PJ. Alternative methods for the control of pain. J Am Vet Med Assoc 2002; 221(2):222–9.
10. AVMA guidelines for complementary and alternative veterinary medicine 2007. Available at: http://www.avma.org/issues/policy/comp_alt_medicine.asp. Accessed June 6, 2010.
11. Lindley S, Cummings M. Essentials of veterinary acupuncture. Ames (IA): Blackwell; 2006.
12. Ma Y, Ma M, Cho ZH. Biomedical acupuncture for pain management: an integrative approach. St Louis (MO): Elsevier; 2005.
13. Dorfer D, Moser M, Bahr F. A medical report from the stone age? Lancet 1999; 354(9183):1023–5.
14. Dorfer L, Moser M, Spindler K, et al. 5200-year-old acupuncture in central Europe? Science 1998;282(5387):242–3.
15. Schoen AM. Veterinary acupuncture ancient art to modern medicine. 2nd edition. Boca Raton (FL): Mosby; 2001.
16. Pyne D, Shenker NG. Demystifying acupuncture. Rheumatology (Oxford) 2008; 47(8):1132–6.
17. Robinson NG. Veterinary acupuncture: an ancient tradition for modern times. Alternative Compl Ther 2007;13(5):259–65.
18. Xie, H. How to use acupuncture for the treatment of osteoarthritis in dogs and cats. Presented at North American Veterinary Conference. Orlando (FL), 2004.
19. Kendall DE. Early understanding of physiology. In: Edwards A, editor. Dao of Chinese medicine: understanding an ancient healing art. Hong Kong: Oxford University Press; 2002.
20. Robinson NG. The need for consistency and comparability of transitional acupuncture points across species. AJTCVM 2006;1(1):14–21.
21. Robinson NG, Pederson J, Burghardt T, et al. Neuroanatomic structure and function of acupuncture points around the eye. AJTCVM 2007;2(1):33–44.
22. Deriu F. Non-nociceptive upper limb afferents modulate masseter muscle EMG activity in man. Exp Brain Res 2002;143:286–94.

23. Dung HC, Clogston CP, Dunn JW. Acupuncture—an anatomical approach. St Louis (MO): CRC Press; 2004. p. 3.
24. Chan SH. What is being stimulated in acupuncture evaluation of the existence of a specific substrate. Neurosci Biobehav Rev 1984;8:25–33.
25. Gaynor JS, Muir WW III. Handbook of veterinary pain management. 2nd edition. St Louis (MO): Mosby; 2009.
26. Zhao Z. Neural mechanism underlying acupuncture analgesia. Prog Neurobiol 2008;85:355–75.
27. Hui K, Nixon E, Vangel MG. Characterization of the "deqi" response in acupuncture. BMC Complement Altern Med 2007;7(33):1–16.
28. Toda K. Afferent nerve characteristics during acupuncture stimulation. Int Congr 2002;1238:49–61.
29. Han JS. Acupuncture: neuropeptide release produced by electrical stimulation of different frequencies. Trends Neurosci 2003;26:17–22.
30. Pomeranz B. Acupuncture analgesia neurophysiological mechanisms. In: Sensory stimulation in pain and diseases—International Congress at the Nobel Forum. Stockholm (Sweden): Karolinska Institute; 1997. p. 7.
31. Han JS. Acupuncture and endorphins. Neurosci Lett 2004;361(1–3):258–61.
32. Moffet HH. How might acupuncture work? A systematic review of physiologic rationales from clinical trials. BMC Complement Altern Med 2006;6:25.
33. Pomeranz B, Paley D. Electroacupuncture hypolgesia is mediated by afferent nerve impulses: an electrophysiological study in mice. Exp Neurol 1979;66: 398–402.
34. Jindal V, Ge A, Mansky PJ. Safety and efficacy of acupuncture in children a review of the evidence. J Pediatr Hematol Oncol 2008;30(6):431–42.
35. Dhond RP, Kettner N, Napadow V. Do the neural correlates of acupuncture and placebo effects differ? Pain 2007;128:8.
36. Kelleher CJ, Filshie J, Burton C, et al. Acupuncture and the treatment if irritable bladder symptoms. Acupunct Med 1994;12(1):9–12.
37. Lundeberg T, Kjartansson J, Samuelson UE. Effect of electrical nerve stimulation on healing ischaemic skin flaps. Lancet 1988;2(8613):712–4.
38. Zhang RX, Lao L, Wang X, et al. Electroacupuncture attenuates inflammation in a rat model. J Altern Complement Med 2005;11(1):135–42.
39. Ezzo JM, Richardson MA, Vickers A. Acupuncture-point stimulation for chemotherapy-induced nausea or vomiting. Cochrane Database Syst Rev 2006;2: CD002285.
40. Li YQ, Zhu B, Rong PJ, et al. Neural mechanisms of acupuncture-modulated gastric motility. World J Gastroenterol 2007;13(5):709–16.
41. Kim HY, Hahm DH, Pyun KH, et al. Effect of traditional acupuncture on proximal colonic motility in conscious dogs. J Vet Med Sci 2006;68(6):603–7.
42. Cho SY, Jahng GH, Park SU, et al. fMRI study of effect on brain activity according to stimulation method at LI11, ST36: painful pressure and acupuncture stimulation of same acupoints. J Altern Complement Med 2010;16(4):489–95.
43. Dhond RP, Yeh C, Park K, et al. Acupuncture modulates resting state connectivity in default and sensorimotor brain networks. Pain 2008;136(3):407–18.
44. Liu JZ, Huang YH, Hand PJ. Effects of dexamethasone on electroacupuncture analgesia and central nervous system metabolism. Acupunct Electrother Res 1988;13(1):9–23.
45. Liu DM, Zhou ZY, Ding Y, et al. Physiologic effects of electroacupuncture combined with intramuscular administration of xylazine to provide analgesia in goats. Am J Vet Res 2009;70(11):1326–32.

46. Yang JW, Jeong SM, Seo KM, et al. Effects of corticosteroid and electroacupuncture on experimental spinal cord injury in dogs. J Vet Sci 2003;4(1):97–101.
47. Eriksson SV, Lundeberg T, Lundeberg S. Interaction of diazepam and naloxone on acupuncture induced pain relief. Am J Chin Med 1991;19(1):1–7.
48. Ernst E, White A. Life threatening adverse reactions after acupuncture? A systematic review. Pain 1997;71:123–6.
49. White A. The safety of acupuncture—evidence from the UK. Acupunct Med 2006; 24:53–7.
50. Acupuncture. NIH Consens Statement 1997;15(5):1–34.
51. Jenkins R. On the state of public health: the annual report of the Chief Medical Officer of the Department of Health for the year 1995. London: HMSO; 1996.
52. Paul-Murphy J, Ludders JW, Robertson SA, et al. The need for a cross-species approach to the study of pain in animals. J Am Vet Med Assoc 2004;224(5): 692–7.
53. Ferguson, B. Practical acupuncture in birds. Presented at Annual Exotics Veterinary Medical Conference. Key West (FL), 2002.
54. Partington M. Avian acupuncture. Probl Vet Med 1992;4(1):212–22.
55. Xie H. What acupuncture can and cannot treat. J Am Anim Hosp Assoc 2006;42: 244–8.
56. Luo D, Liu S, Xie X, et al. Electroacupuncture at acupoint ST-36 promotes contractility of distal colon via a cholinergic pathway in conscious rats. Dig Dis Sci 2008;53:689–93.
57. Kelly RB. Acupuncture for pain. Am Fam Physician 2009;80(5):481–4.
58. Merritt AM, Xie H, Lester GD, et al. Evaluation of a method to experimentally induce colic in horses and the effects of acupuncture applied at the Guan-yuan-shu (similar to BL-21) acupoint. Am J Vet Res 2002;63(7):1006–11.
59. Xie H, Colahan P, Ott EA. Evaluation of electroacupuncture treatment of horses with signs of chronic thoracolumbar pain. J Am Vet Med Assoc 2005;227(2): 281–6.
60. Cui KM, Li WM, Gao X. Electroacupuncture relieves chronic visceral hyperalgesia in rats. Neurosci Lett 2005;376(20):20–3.
61. Goddard G. Short term pain reduction with acupuncture treatment for chronic orofacial pain patients. Med Sci Monit 2005;11(2):CR71–4.
62. White A, Tough E, Cummings M. A review of acupuncture clinical trials indexed during 2005. Acupunct Med 2006;24(1):39–49.
63. Yin J, Chen JD. Gastrointestinal motility disorders and acupuncture. Auton Neurosci 2010. [Epub ahead of print]. DOI:10.1016/j.autneu.2010.03.007.
64. Niu WX, He GD, Liu H, et al. Effects and probable mechanisms of electroacupuncture at the Zusanli point on upper gastrointestinal motility in rabbits. J Gastroenterol Hepatol 2007;22:1683–9.
65. Lloret L, Hayhoe S. A tale of two foxes—case reports: 1. Radial nerve paralysis treated with acupuncture in a wild fox 2. Acupuncture in a fox with aggressive and obsessive behaviour. Acupunct Med 2005;23(4):190–5.
66. Crouch MA. Egg binding and hind limb paralysis in an African penguin—a case report. Acupunct Med 2009;27(1):36–8.
67. Scognamillo-Szabó MV, Santos AL, Olegário MM, et al. Acupuncture for locomotor disabilities in a South American red-footed tortoise (Geochelone carbonaria)—a case report. Acupunct Med 2008;26(4):243–7.
68. Lao L, Wong RH, Wynn RL. Electroacupuncture reduces morphine-induced emesis in ferrets: a pilot study. J Altern Complement Med 1995;1(3):257–61.

Index

Note: Page numbers of article titles are in **boldface** type.

A

Acetaminophen (paracetamol), for pain, in ferrets, 108–109
    in rodents, 86–87
Acetic acid test (AAT), in pain model, in amphibians, 36–37, 39
Acupoints, in acupuncture, 145–146, 150
Acupuncture, for zoologic companion animals, **141–154**
    acupoints in, 145–146, 150
    CAVM vs., 142
    conditions commonly considered for, 151
    contraindications for, 147
    critics of, 141–142
    definition of, 143
    history of, 144–145
    legality in U.S., 142–143
    mechanism of action, 145–147
      pain and, 147–148
    need for, 141
    patient selection for, 150–151
    safety of, 147
    summary overview of, 141–142, 151
    traditional Chinese, 143–145, 150
    training for, 143, 147
    unique aspects of, anatomic, 150
      behavioral, 148–150
  transpositional, 145
α2-Adrenergic agonists, for pain, in ferrets, 110, 112
    in rabbits, 100
    in reptiles, 53, 56
Adrenergic system, stress and, in fish, 22
Adrenocorticotropic hormone (ACTH), stress and, in fish, 22
Adverse effects, of analgesia, detection of, in controlled clinical trials, 4
Algesiometric model, of pain, in amphibians, 36
Allometric analysis, in pharmacokinetic studies, 10–14
    scaling of, 13–14
Allometric scaling, application of, 13–14
α2-Adrenergic agonists, for pain, in ferrets, 110, 112
    in rabbits, 100
    in reptiles, 53, 56
Amphibians, analgesia in, **33–44**
    acupuncture as, 148–149
    clinical applications of, 38–39
    neuroanatomy and, 34–36

Vet Clin Exot Anim 14 (2011) 155–177
doi:10.1016/S1094-9194(10)00137-4
1094-9194/11/$ – see front matter © 2011 Elsevier Inc. All rights reserved.

vetexotic.theclinics.com

Moving?

Make sure your subscription moves with you!

To notify us of your new address, find your **Clinics Account Number** (located on your mailing label above your name), and contact customer service at:

Email: journalscustomerservice-usa@elsevier.com

800-654-2452 (subscribers in the U.S. & Canada)
314-447-8871 (subscribers outside of the U.S. & Canada)

Fax number: 314-447-8029

Elsevier Health Sciences Division
Subscription Customer Service
3251 Riverport Lane
Maryland Heights, MO 63043

*To ensure uninterrupted delivery of your subscription, please notify us at least 4 weeks in advance of move.

Moving?

Printed and bound by CPI Group (UK) Ltd, Croydon, CR0 4YY

14/10/2024

01773702-0003